THE BALANCING ACT

How to Live a Wholesome Life

by
Samantha Baird

THE BALANCING ACT
How to Live a Wholesome Life

Copyright © 2013 by Samantha Baird

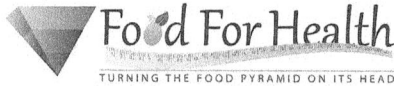

Food For Health
TURNING THE FOOD PYRAMID ON ITS HEAD

All Rights Reserved.

ISBN: 978-0-9923830-0-8

TABLE OF
CONTENTS

DAY 1:
Changing Your Mindset

"It's not the strongest of the species that survives, nor the most intelligent, but the one most adaptable to change."

~ **Charles Darwin** ~

I F YOU'RE READING THIS book, there is probably something about your health you're not happy about. Maybe you're in pain, unhappy with your weight, or you're sick and tired of being sick and tired. No doubt you know others who are also struggling with their health, but you're here reading this book, and it's likely they are not.

What is the difference between you and them?

Well, if you're reading this book it should mean that you're willing to make some changes. It should mean that you're willing to evaluate your life, take stock of your habits, examine your lifestyle, and consider making some changes. Perhaps even big changes.

> **TIP:** *As you progress through the book, you may encounter terminology unfamiliar to you. A list of helpful terms with definitions is provided in Appendix C for your reference.*

Welcome to Day 1 of your new journey. This phase of your life has the potential to be different from everything you have ever experienced before today. However this will only be true if you commit to reading the words, absorbing the knowledge to your brain and the wisdom to your heart, and begin to make the necessary changes that give you a different life than what you have already experienced.

Remember—you're here right now because you are unhappy where you are. Something about your life displeases you. To have a different life means to make changes, and it needs to begin today. Not tomorrow.

○ HOW TO USE THIS BOOK

If you've been dealing with health problems for a long time, you are probably tired or angry. You've tried different things to fix your health and they didn't work, and it frustrated you. You want this time to be different, but maybe you are not even sure you have the strength to try again. I understand, and I've been there too.

This book is not intended to be an exhaustive resource. Rather it is intended to keep things simple by giving you nutrition and other information in bite-size, easily digestible pieces, so that you can quickly absorb what you need to know and move on. Additional resources are available to expand your knowledge, as well as assist you with shopping and building routines.

The good news is that the content in this book is flexible and easy to implement over time and at your own pace. We will do this by viewing each change as a mini commitment. Here is your first commitment.

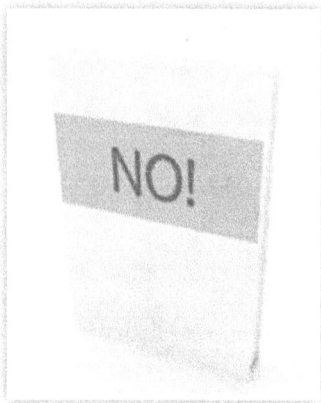

Commitment #1: *Read through this entire book.*

The book has been broken up into "days" for your journey, but these "days" are a recommendation, not a requirement. Think of them as fluid. If it takes you a single day to complete Day 1, that is fine. If it takes you a week to complete Day 1, that is okay too. Just stop, close your eyes, and make a commitment to yourself that you will read the entire book "cover to cover", a little more every day.

○ SIMPLE STEPS

First things first. We will tackle areas of frustration in your life by completing the following steps:

- Identifying bad habits
- Rejecting bad habits
- Choosing good habits

We will apply these simple steps throughout this book, and it will change your life. It's okay if you do not believe it yet--just stick with your original commitment to read it. That's all you have to do.

Identify Bad Habits

> **TIP:** *If you would like coaching during your health and life journey, contact certified food coach Samantha Baird at www.food4health.com.au for coaching options and resources.*

The first step to changing anything you are unhappy with is figuring out what you're doing wrong. Forget about assigning blame or pointing the finger at other people or situations. The point is, you may not be able to control everything about how you got to where you are at, but you *can* change the things you have control of—so focus on that. Don't stress over the rest.

To identify bad habits, you will be asked questions to consider what you might be experiencing in that area. You will need to do some soul searching, and maybe even talk to family or friends who know you well (sometimes you find out some pretty interesting things when you do this). You don't need to ask the opinion of those you do not trust; just stick with those who know you best and love you.

Reject Bad Habits

Once you have identified bad habits in your life, you will need to make a commitment to reject those things which are hurting you or which you know are bad for you. Don't keep rubbish in your life; it acts like a slow poison that leaches into everything. Toss it and go!

Remember, we are going to tackle these issues one at a time—not all at once. Don't stress. Baby steps only.

Choose Good Habits

Once you have made a choice to reject a bad habit, there is one more step to take and it is critical—you must replace the bad habit with a good habit. It is not enough to simply reject bad habits; you must replace those behaviours with something new and healthy for you.

The choices we make in our lives fill up a hole of some type—people we love, things we love, jobs, careers, and yes, even our hobbies or our addictions. They feed a 'need' in our personalities. You cannot leave the hole empty or something else equally unhealthy may take its place. It's why ex-smokers often gain weight—they replace their nicotine addiction with food addiction.

We will talk about healthy options to form good habits. You will get support each step of the way, and you will live differently. And you will change—one step at a time.

○ HELP FOR BUILDING GOOD HABITS

Throughout the book there will be references to specialized handouts, lists, cheat sheets, and other resources for you to use at your discretion. They are intended to be flexible and useful for implementing changes to your life; think of them as tools to help you on your way.

These resources are referenced throughout the book but found in Appendix A for easy reference.

However, the most important asset you can have on your side is a positive attitude. A good attitude helps you to cope with stressful events and improves your immune system[1]—both benefits have a positive impact to your health.

We've all heard it said that a positive attitude can change your entire outlook on life and it's true. It's important that whatever your past that you face the future with a smile on your face and believe that life can be better. You can do this!

If you are not there yet, just continue reading the book. Give yourself time—but not a free pass. A more hopeful perspective on life can come, but it's also easy to allow blame and bitterness from previous failures to cloud your judgment; therefore, do your best *now* to be open minded to changing your outlook on life as you go. It's just another part of making the journey, but the journey goes by quicker and easier with joy in your heart! Don't overthink each step. Once you understand your next course of action, take it and then read on to discover what's next.

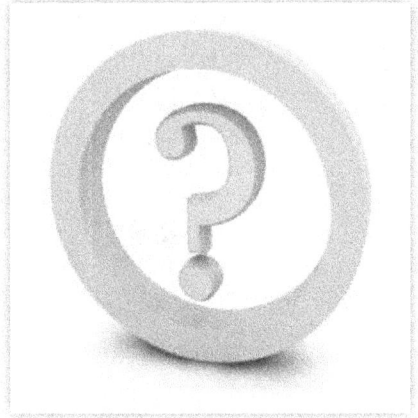

○ WHAT TO AVOID

While you are taking those first important baby steps on your journey, it is important to avoid people who might discourage you, regardless of their possible good intentions. People will naysay your efforts for a lot of reasons:

- They've seen you try before and fail, and they want to protect you from repeat failure
- They don't understand your motivation to change
- They believe you are imagining or exaggerating your symptoms
- They're jealous of your willingness and ability to change

Do not listen to the negative voices of others. Let them know that you don't need their negativity in your life, and if they continue to push your buttons, consider avoiding them for a little while. If they can't support you in your efforts, then they are a distraction.

To improve your circumstances is going to take time. It is time that is well spent and an investment in your future—as well as the lives of those you might bless—but you might feel a bit fragile emotionally and mentally right now. If you do, don't feel the slightest bit of guilt about avoiding those whose actions would ultimately harm your goals. Move forward—at least for a time—and 'love' who they are from a distance.

◯ THE BIG SECRET

There is one big secret to all of this. One thing that is a huge game changer as you move forward. It's so important that it draws the line in the sand between success and failure!

The answer can be found throughout the pages of this book, but just in case you don't figure it out, I will lay it all out in black and white later. For right now, just read.

DAY 2:
Nutrition

DAY 2 OF YOUR journey will begin with a study on the basics of nutrition. There is a lot of information floating around out there and we all know the internet has turned into a real mess, in particular for issues relating to health, exercise, dietary concerns, illness, etc.

My best suggestion to you is to wipe the slate clean. Learn everything new from the ground up, because almost everything you know is going to be wrong, or some sort of mixture of right and wrong. It will be easier for you to simply start fresh—and so we'll start with the basics.

A final comment before we start. You will read the use of the term "diet" or "dietary" throughout this section—please understand the usage of this term to mean a long-term eating plan, or an established set of food choices. This term does *not* refer to fad or short-term eating plans, which are bad for your health and do not succeed in helping with long-term health goals. We're in this for the long haul. You will never need—or want—to 'diet' again!

○ WHAT IS NUTRITION?

You already know you need energy to survive. That energy is produced from the foods you eat, which are used as raw materials for growth and energy. However, not all foods are created equal. Some foods are clearly better choices than others, and a little bit of knowledge helps you make the right choices.

The impact of nutrition on your health cannot be overstated, and we'll research that in more detail. The good news is that no matter how you've eaten before today, you can change your life dramatically by changing what you eat. You cannot do this with a fad diet, but you can do it with a long-term focus on good dietary choices. Be encouraged that even if you have been eating poorly your entire life—if you grew up eating fried foods every day, for example—it is never too late to make a positive change.

It is true that the longer you have eaten poorly, the more negative the impact it can have on your life. However, you already know it's had a negative impact—it's why you're reading this book. So toss aside the negative thoughts that might naturally occur here and zone in on the fact that things can improve beginning today. Beginning *now*.

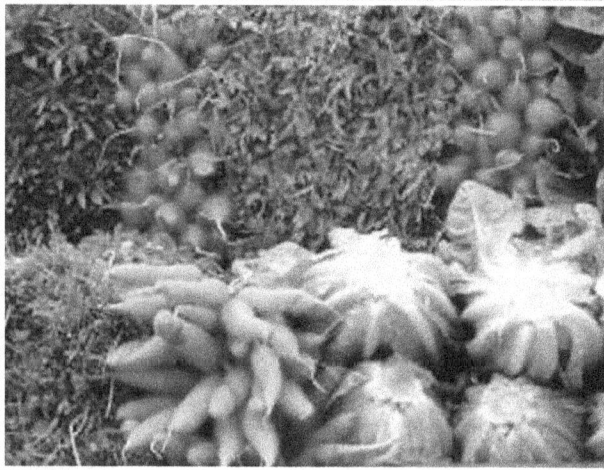

Aside from the health improvements, there are other benefits to living a healthier lifestyle. You can expect your quality of life to improve as stress has less of an impact because your immune system is not overtaxed. Making certain food choices can even simplify your life, reduce decision making (which eases stress), and have the ability to fight the degenerative effects of aging.[2]

There are additional reasons to enjoy living a healthy lifestyle, but we'll dig into them more later. Just know that with good nutrition comes many blessings—that's something you can look forward to.

○ NUTRITION BASICS

Water itself is a basic nutrient and is essential to survival and body processes. Two thirds of your body is water and you should be drinking your 3 - 4 liters of purified water every day. In addition, drinking purified water helps you avoid accumulating excess fluoride in your body which studies have linked to damaged reproductive systems, early onset of puberty, neurotoxicity, impacts to thyroid function, the development of arthritis, and more.[3] I highly recommend you invest in a ceramic water filter that will remove the fluoride from tap water.

Now on to food! The food you eat can be broken into two main nutritional categories: macronutrients and micronutrients.

Macronutrients

Macronutrient foods are your carbohydrates, fats, and proteins. Carbs are broken down into individual fructose, galactose, or glucose units. Your body chooses glucose as its primary source for energy, because it is easy to burn. Glucose is usually sourced from carbohydrates; however, if you eat too many carbs, your body is very efficient at storing them as fat in your adipose tissues (under-the-skin fat). If you do not overeat on your carbs, your body can also get energy by producing glucose from protein through a biological process known as gluconeogenesis.

REFERENCE: See *Identify Your Food Habits*

Fats are divided into four categories: saturated, trans, polyunsaturated, and monounsaturated. The two fats to generally avoid are saturated and trans fats, which should be consumed in limited quantities due to their negative impact on cholesterol levels. Saturated fats tend to be animal based, are solid at room temperature, and trans fats are processed, or synthetic fats, created when foods are fried. However, some fats are beneficial, which we will discuss in more detail later.

Micronutrients

Micronutrients are the vitamins and minerals you absorb. They act as co-enzymes which perform like energy boosts to help your body's chemical reactions happen faster. Your body needs requires varying amounts of each, and having too much or too little can impact your health.

In addition, antioxidants also help your body. They are found in the phytochemicals (phyto is Greek for 'plant') of vegies and fruits, and they help your body fight off some of the damage caused by pollution, smoke, sun exposure, and poor dietary choices. Some antioxidants even have an anti-inflammatory and antihistamine impact on your body, so while you may only need antioxidants in minimal doses, they can have a big impact on the quality of your health.

○ WHAT HAVE YOU BEEN EATING?

We all know that eating lots of fruits and vegies is better for us than eating lots of fast food and processed foods, yet we still don't eat the vegies that we should. Sodas are harmful—most of us drink them anyway. On a regular basis, most of us continue to make poor dietary choices, and these choices are slowly hurting us, and even leading us to a premature death.

To change this unhealthy cycle, let's consider our own eating habits. I warned you before that we would review our habits, because you need to be honest with *you* about what you are doing. As humans, we're good at lying to ourselves about touchy subject matters, such as how we eat. We tend to think we eat pretty well with just an occasional gap in making good choices. Sometimes that is the truth, and sometimes it's not entirely accurate.

Let's take a few minutes to evaluate how you eat.

Identify Your Food Habits

To better understand how your eating practices may have played a part in your current health situation, let's look at your previous eating habits. To do that, print "Identify Your Food Habits" and fill it out.

REFERENCE	LOCATION
Identify Your Food Habits	96

Food For Health

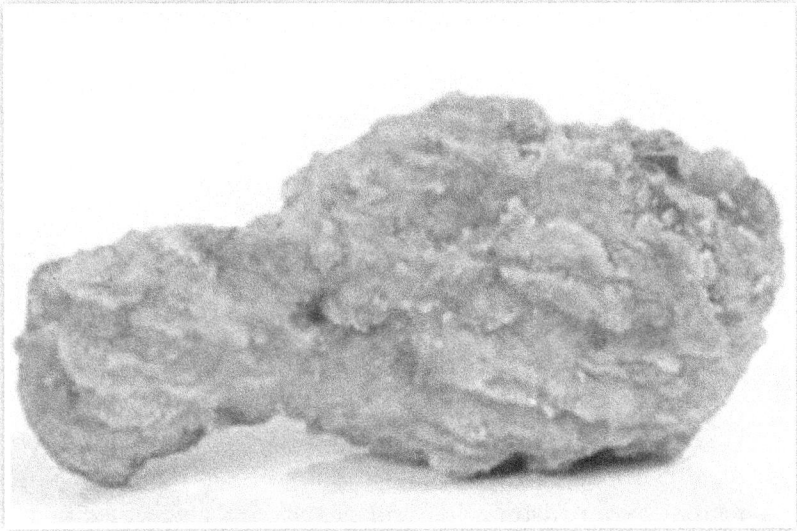

This worksheet will help you examine:

- past food choices from your childhood
- who taught you what you know about nutrition
- what you regard as acceptable food choices
- your current list of health complaints

This may take you a day to fill out, or a week; it's up to you. Once you have completed the worksheet, if you are already willing to make changes to your dietary habits right now, you can continue forward and complete the Nutrition chapter of this book. In other words, you can move forward while you are simultaneously examining your dietary past so you can learn from it.

If, however, you are not willing to make any changes to how you eat, then you should thoroughly complete this step before moving any further. It is important that you understand that there are things about food you can control, and that *you* are responsible for those things. This is not an attempt to burden you or fill you with guilt; instead, it's intended to empower you to learn from the past and make better choices in the future. Learning from our mistakes is what life is all about, and we've all been there!

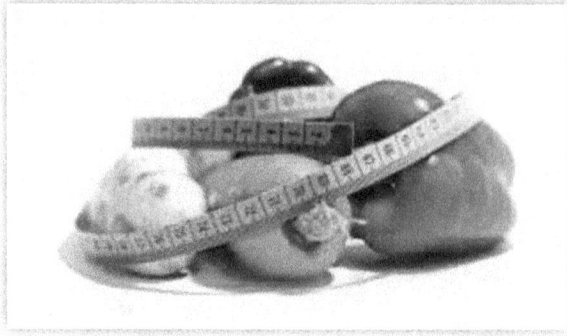

Reject Your Bad Food Habits

Once you have completed your "Identify Your Food Habits" worksheet, it's time to consider what you've written. Was it enlightening? Did you learn some facts about your history you had never considered or didn't know about?

Most of us find that we pieced together ideas about nutrition from our parents or other caregivers. They probably learnt from their parents or caregivers, and in the end, some of them may not have been the most informed about good dietary choices. They simply did what most people do—they made do with what they knew. They simply didn't know any better.

Living in the information age—as well as the age of obesity—we know now that something has gone very wrong. Either our understanding of good nutrition has been incorrect and is catching up with us, or something has changed about the food sources we consume—or perhaps more likely, the answer is a combination of the two. We'll talk more about this in our consultations, but for now, we won't be derailed by looking at the universal 'why'.

What is important is *you*. Now that you've examined your past, you know that you've made some mistakes. You've made some bad food choices. Everybody does. Nutrition is a skill you must learn; you aren't born knowing all the facts. What you can do right now is reject those bad dietary habits you've formed, accept that what you knew about food was probably a mixture of right and wrong, and that you can learn to make better choices for your future.

Most people make dietary decisions that directly contradict good choices, and many seem to think the body is resilient enough to tolerate their bad choices without worry. However, my belief is that not only are these serious choices, but these poor choices are literally pushing people toward an early grave. It does matter to your body if you choose to consume sugar, toxic oils, processed foods, dairy, and grain, and the consequences are severe!

Choosing Good Food Habits

To improve your life, it's important that we replace the bad eating habits with good ones. When you make good choices, you'll begin to feel better and have more energy. You may also discover that you've been struggling with deficiencies or food intolerances, and these have also impacted your health. If you weren't aware of these deficiencies or intolerances, you couldn't do anything about them—but with knowledge comes power.

The truth is that you *do* have control over what you choose to eat, and you *can* protect your family from many of the additives and preservatives in food by making smart choices. This is where making the hard choices as a mum or dad come into play. You have the power to say no and give your children a future of good health. As you read through this chapter, you will learn more about how important your decisions will be regarding vegies, grain, dairy, and more—which this brings us to the next commitment!

Commitment #2: *Choose an eating plan for you and your family and stick with it for 6 months.*

It's my hope that you will stick with this new plan for the rest of your life, but for now—just agree to 6 months.

The upcoming sections will lay out options for positive eating choices that are healthy and provide beneficial nutrition to your body. It's important that you carefully read through the options, choose the one that works best for you—and then stick with it.

○ WHEN TO EAT

There is a fairly common school of thought circulating in health circles right now—including by medical professionals—that you should eat every 3 to 4 hours per day, for a total of around 6 meals.

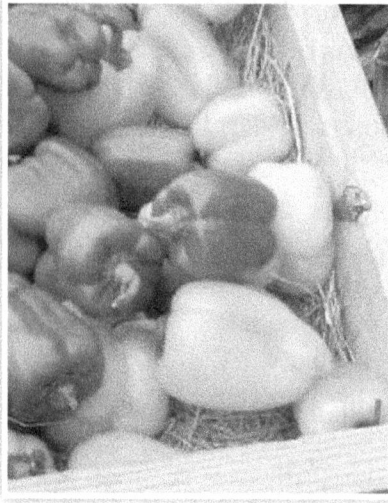

There are a couple problems with this concept. The first issue is that this type of eating requires a huge amount of portion control. The simple fact is most people will not estimate calories accurately enough to prevent accidental overeating.

The second problem is that there is little historical example of people eating that way. Instead, people ate when they were hungry and when they were able to acquire food.

I teach people to eat 2 - 3 large meals per day, and *to wait to eat until hungry*. If you wait to eat when hunger pain strikes, you can be confident you are not eating too soon, thereby helping to prevent consuming too many calories over the course of the day.

In addition, occasional fasting can be healthy for the body. I recommend fasting at least once per month. Also, our bodies naturally fast every night while we sleep, with peak digestion occurring between 3:00 – 5:00am. If you control your eating the evening before, you can take maximum advantage of your nightly fast; it's critical for giving your body a chance to properly digest and clear out all the food eaten the previous day.

Now that we've talked about *how often* to put food into your body, let's talk about *what* food should go into your body.

○ WHAT TO EAT

To apply good nutrition, we'll study two different dietary options, or food plans. For those who can embrace the restrictions, a strictly raw food eating plan is the ideal choice. For people who 'can't live without' meat, I recommend the RPP plan. However, the overall rule of thumb is: anything that grows out of the ground is good, anything with a heartbeat is good, but anything out of a box should be avoided.

> **TIP:** *Chop your fresh vegies and store in jars in the fridge — that's one less thing to do during the week, and they can be stored up to five days!*

Read below to get a better understanding of these two fantastic roads to enjoying healthy food!

REFERENCE	LOCATION
Raw Foods Eating Plan Breakdown	97
Green Vegies article	http://www.food4health.com.au/green-vegetables/
Raw Vegie Protein Cheat Sheet	100
Blender Review	102
Smoothie Cleanse FAQ	104
How to Make a Salad a Complete Meal	106
Recipes	Appendix B

Option A: Raw Foods Only

For those who are willing, a raw foods eating lifestyle can be the fastest track back to good health. Raw food eating consists of organic raw vegies, fruits, sprouts, roots, nuts, and seeds, all of which have not been cooked above 46 degrees Celsius. Obviously simple chopped fruits and vegies are allowed, but you would probably get bored eventually without any variety! There are innumerable, flavourful recipe options for preparing raw food dishes, and these more creative food choices are typically prepared using a quality blender, food processor, and dehydrator.

Raw foods are considered healthy because they are the most pure, whole foods we can eat. This dietary plan also includes living foods which are made up of raw foods that have been soaked and left to sprout, releasing the enzymes in the food.

Cooked foods are chemically altered by heat which can impact their nutritional value. By contrast, living and raw food offers the best use of the natural properties of fruits and vegies to give your body the most wholesome nutrition possible.

Food For Health
TURNING THE FOOD PYRAMID ON ITS HEAD

Some foods within the raw foods plan do require cooking, such as legumes and potatoes; however, those choices should be kept at a minimum. To aid in the digestive breakdown of foods, a better option is to blend or juice your foods to produce the affect of bursting open the foods cells—which aid in easier digestion—without applying high heat to foods resulting in a loss of nutrients.[4]

Your typical day as a 'raw foodie' might look something like this:

- Breakfast—creamy fruit and vegie smoothie with super foods and a nut milk base or homemade granola with coconut yogurt and fresh fruit
- Lunch—Nori or lettuce/kale leaf wraps filled with avocado sprouts, grated carrots, greens, and tomatoes (make several) or raw sushi filled with raw cauliflower or parsnip rice, plus chopped vegies, rolled and served with wheat free tamari
- Snack—a few bananas, protein balls, handful of nuts, or some fresh fruit
- Dinner—a complete meal salad (refer to "How to Make a Salad a Complete Meal") or zucchini noodles or coconut laksa
- Dessert—homemade ice cream, pudding, or mousse

> TIP: *Prepare two or three salads at the start of the week so that you can easily pack and go!*

Refer to the references below for more information.

REFERENCE	LOCATION
Raw Foods Eating Plan Breakdown	97
Green Vegies article	http://www.food4health.com.au/green-vegetables/
Raw Vegie Protein Cheat Sheet	100
Blender Review	102
Smoothie Cleanse FAQ	104
How to Make a Salad a Complete Meal	106
9 Day "Get Started" Meal Plan	111
Recipes	Appendix B

Option B: Raw Plus Paleo (RPP)

If you've been eating a traditional meat diet in the past and you are unwilling to give up meat, you will most likely consider switching to my Raw Plus Paleo (RPP) plan. This flexible option allows for a balance between raw foods and smart meat choices.

The concept behind the Paleo 'diet' is that you eat from the food groups our Paleolithic era ancestors would have eaten, who would have been primarily hunter-gatherers. Therefore Paleo acceptable foods consist of fresh fruits, vegies, seeds, nuts, oils, seafood, eggs, and grass-fed, free-range meats.

Paleo excludes dairy, cereal grains, refined sugars, potatoes, salt, processed foods, and refined vegetable oils.

On the RPP plan you eat vegies following the Raw Food Plan 1 – 2 days each week and Paleo the remainder of the week; however, all meals should include 50% and up raw food components. Organic, free-range chicken eggs, as well as fish, can be eaten as a healthy option at any meal.

The goal is to stay conscious of using vegetables to remain alkaline while following a healthy meat-eating diet (read up on alkalinity in the "Acid Vs. Alkaline" section).

Your typical day might look something like this:

- Breakfast—(stick with raw foods for breakfast) try the Green Pancakes recipe (Appendix B) topped with fresh fruit and freshly squeezed juice
- Lunch—baked meatballs with a salad, zucchini slice or mini quiches, bolognaise muffins, or soup, or chicken salad
- Snack—same as raw food options, but you could also toss in a treat like Paleo cookies
- Dinner—steak and salad, roast and vegetable, zucchini bolognaise, or crispy skin salmon
- Dessert—homemade ice cream, pudding, or mousse

You don't need to count calories with this plan either—just make sure every meal is at least half raw foods.

Refer to the references below for more information.

> **Caution:** *Avoid pre-packaged gluten free products where possible as they are filled with unhealthy preservatives and may contain soy products!*

REFERENCE	LOCATION
Elimination Diet for Gluten	112
Gluten Free Ingredients List	114
Gluten Free Shopping List	117

○ OTHER FOOD CHOICES TO CONSIDER

Once you've chosen which food plan best fits your health and lifestyle, there are still other food choices to consider. The information below provides you with additional detail on beneficial foods, as well as how to avoid foods that could harm you.

Coeliac and Gluten Intolerance

To open this section, I will begin with a startling statement: *I believe that all grains are bad. I also believe that 95% of people are gluten intolerant and suffer from intestinal permeability.* This perspective might seem extreme or shocking to some, but the consequences of grains are huge and should be heavily considered when having health problems.

If you are unfamiliar with coeliac disease or gluten intolerance, to summarize, both groups cannot consume wheat, barley (including malt), rye, triticale, kamut, spelt, bulgur, durum wheat, farina, graham, semolina, and sometimes oats. The difference between the two conditions is that coeliac disease is an autoimmune disorder, but for both health conditions there is no 'cure', and the only healthy alternative is to avoid all forms of gluten for life.

The consequences of eating grains when you cannot digest them are far reaching, resulting in systemic inflammation and a variety of health issues. Here are a few problems—and these are really just the tip of the iceberg:

- depression, in particular for those who are also obese (adipose fat tissue releases IL-1 cytokines[5] which block the production of serotonin 5-HT, the 'feel good' hormone [6])
- intestinal permeability, i.e., leaky gut, where the walls and villi of the bowel are damaged allowing microbes, toxins, waste, and undigested food to pass through them, causing an immune reaction[7]
- chronic inflammation, in particular when associated with highly refined starchy foods, and which is tied to "a myriad of degenerative, modern diseases including arthritis, allergies, asthma, cardiovascular disease, bone loss, emotional imbalance and even cancer."[8]

Grains are actually seeds. We soak seeds in order to remove or reduce the phytic acid on them—which is poisonous—and we attempt to digest what is left over. Seeds protect themselves so they can eventually germinate. Unfortunately, our grains are ground so fine that the seed's protection is removed and we consume all the stuff in the seed we should not. The exposure to the harmful contents in seeds is exposed to the villa in our colons; the villa are the finger-like projections that line the walls of our colon and absorb the nutrients from our food. Grains shoot through the villa in our colons leaving bullet-like holes behind which cause the intestinal permeability mentioned above. The result is inflammation and chronic disease.

In addition, many people are unaware that serotonin, the 'feel good' hormone (neurotransmitter), is produced in the gut, and when our digestive system is impaired we can experience depression due to poor bowel health.[9] In fact, these neurons associated with the enteric nervous system in our digestive tract are informally referred to as our 'second brain'[10] and perform many similar functions to our 'primary' brain, but specific to regulating the gut. In addition, wheat proteins, or peptides, have shown to produce "opioid-like activity in in vitro tests", meaning that wheat can actually produce a chemically addictive reaction in our bodies, similar to opiates.[11] Yes, it is true—you can become addicted to bread!

> **Caution:** *Avoid overcooking animal proteins as this will destroy the amino acids in the food!*

Hopefully the true impact of dealing with digestive problems is becoming a little clearer. *The health of our gut is critical to our overall health.* If we choose to eat foods that inflame our gut, we will face significant health consequences.

Refer to the references below for more information.

Fermented Foods

Fermented foods are food items preserved using lactic acid to produce the bacteria lactobacilli, which offer probiotic benefits. Basically, the food is captured in a state between fresh and spoiled. It sounds a little off, but fermented foods have been popular in most cultures throughout human history and offer people many benefits today.

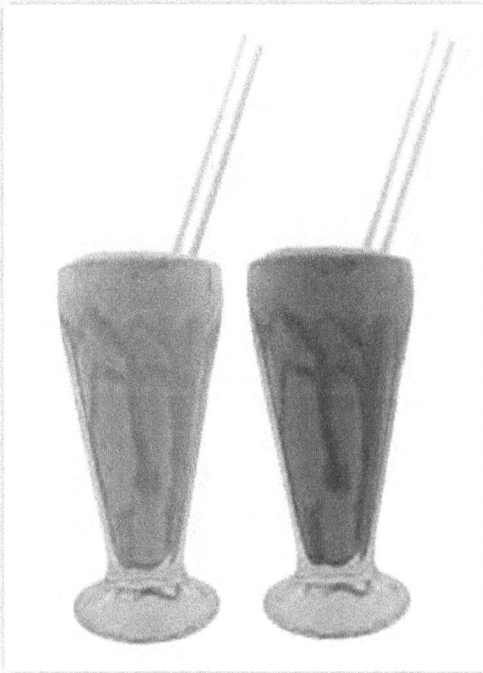

In fact, if you suffer from any sort of digestive ailment, fermented foods are your best friend! Why? Well, fermented foods contain living organisms, i.e., bacteria, helpful for rebuilding the good bacteria in your gut in order to heal from the ravaging effects of bacterial imbalances, including the consumption of gluten, antibiotics, and more. These food enzymes are essential for our very life. If we didn't have them in our gut, we would die, and when we lack enough good bacteria or flora to digest our food, we can get very sick.

Helpful fermented foods include yogurt, kefir, kombucha, kimchi, and sauerkraut.

We'll talk more about preparing fermented foods in Day 3!

REFERENCE	LOCATION
Protein Powder Alternatives	121
Raw Vegie Protein Cheat Sheet	100
Blender Review	102
Smoothie Cleanse FAQ	104

Protein

Protein is essential for many of your bodily processes, including building and repairing tissue, as well as making hormones and enzymes.

Food should always be chosen with protein count in mind. Not only is adequate protein helpful for energy levels and sustaining blood sugars, but choosing vegies with complete protein (or whole protein) are particularly important, as they contain all nine of the essential amino acids required for optimum health. These essential amino acids, and their associated protein levels, are:

- Leucine (55 mg/g)
- Lysine (51 mg/g)
- Phenylalanine + Tyrosine (47 mg/g)
- Valine (32 mg/g)
- Threonine (27 mg/g)
- Isoleucine (25 mg/g)
- Methionine + Cystine (25 mg/g)
- Histidine (18 mg/g)
- Tryptophan (7 mg/g)

When you eat a meal containing proportionate levels of each of the nine essential amino acids, you form a complete protein chain, similar to the linking chains in a necklace. You can research the amino acids in plants if you are curious; however, to keep it simple, it is known that most animal proteins are complete proteins, and many vegetable proteins are complete, with a few exceptions where they lack in one or two amino acids. Therefore, this problem is easily resolved for raw food eating by simply consuming a variety of plant sources each meal to ensure all amino acids are present.

Another protein source that many will often turn to is dairy; however, I highly recommend my clients avoid dairy for a variety of reasons. First, most diary is contaminated by antibiotics and growth hormones fed to the animals. Also, animal dairy is often poor quality due to the animal receiving a poor diet or living under stressful conditions. It's also been determined that most adults lack the enzyme (lactase) required to properly digest cow dairy (lactose); the result is that it often ends up a sour mess that disturbs the digestive tract of many individuals, sometimes even clogging up the liver as it attempts to filter it.[12] When a recipe requires milk, the best option is to choose non-dairy substitutes, such as almond or coconut milk. If you do choose to keep dairy in your diet, source raw dairy straight from an organic farmer instead.

Soy is another protein source I strongly recommend my clients not consume. Soy can be found in whole bean form as well as seen on labels, such as soy lecithin. All soy products should be avoided. The short explanation on this is that soy mimics estrogen, which therefore messes with women's hormones and lowers men's testosterone levels. Depending on age, sex, and other genetic factors, it can have a varying negative impact for the person consuming it. In fact, around two thousand years ago, monks in the Orient actually consumed soy by choice in order to assist with their sexual abstinence due to its known ability to lower libidos (via reducing testosterone levels)!

In short, avoid soy at all costs and check labels to ensure you are not consuming food containing soy.

Many people who are attempting to live healthier lifestyles often turn to protein powder shakes for boosting their protein levels, improving their exercise recovery, etc. These products may claim they are healthy on the fancy packaging, but they often contain toxins (sugars or other unhealthy carbs) that spike your blood sugar and contain gluten. Instead, stick to healthy smoothies

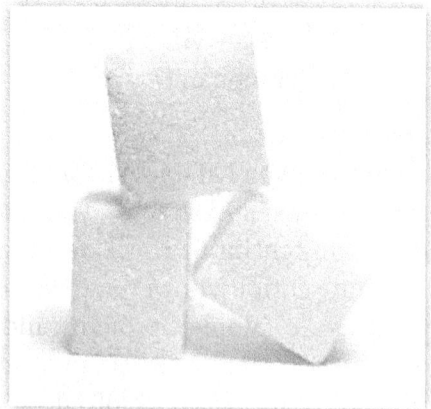

and natural vegie proteins, and avoid the artificial or fake sweeteners, and unhealthy by-products in these items.

Finally, there is a word of caution. While adequate protein is important, there is no need to overindulge. It is possible to eat more protein than your body can adequately process and it can stress your body. Shoot for healthy protein counts and not sky high; the Ministry of Health recommends 64g for men and 46g for women daily.[13]

Refer to the references below for more information.

Good Carbs, Bad Carbs, and Sugars

Carbohydrates are always in the middle of heated health debates. To some, it is an ugly word—they think instant weight gain! Are they good for you or bad for you? Ignore the arguing and simplify your life by not grouping all carbs into one category and evaluating their merit overall. Instead, be aware there are better carb choices while there are some carbs that you would do better to avoid entirely.

Good quality carb choices include those high in fiber, such as dehydrated fruits, and fresh fruits and vegies. Due to their high fiber content, these carbs are absorbed more slowly by the body, and therefore, you avoid an unhealthy spike in your blood sugar (repeat or regular spikes in blood sugar can eventually lead to insulin resistance and Type 2 diabetes).[14]

Bad carb choices include those with sugars or refined flours, such as sugars (sucrose, or table sugar), drink powders, cereals, flours, salad dressings, and jam. These carbs will spike your blood sugar, and should be avoided.[14]

In Australia there has been a lot of media coverage on how bad sugars are for us. Anti-sugar campaigners, author's David Gillespie and Sara Wilson, strongly advise to give it up completely.

Professor Robert Lutsig, an American paediatric endocrinologist at the University of California, labeled sugar as toxic and called it to be taxed the same as alcohol. Lutsig says the sugars added to processed foods are causing metabolic syndrome, conditions such as high blood pressure, and carrying too much fat around the abdomen, as well as high blood sugar, which increases your risk of Type 2 diabetes, stroke, and heart disease. You'll read more on this later.

Here are some facts regarding the Australian obesity crises, from the Monash University website:

- "Fourteen million Australians are overweight or obese.
- More than five million Australians are obese (BMI = 30 kg/m^2).
- If weight gain continues at current levels, by 2025, close to 80% of all Australian adults and a third of all children will be overweight or obese.
- Obesity has overtaken smoking as the leading cause of premature death and illness in Australia.
- Obesity has become the single biggest threat to public health in Australia.
- On basis of present trends we can predict that by the time they reach the age of 20 our kids will have a shorter life expectancy than earlier generations simply because of obesity.
- Australians reporting heart, stroke, and vascular diseases aged 15 years and over were much more likely to be classified as overweight or obese than those without heart, stroke, and vascular disease (65% compared with 51%).
- Health disorders in children like type 2 diabetes, high blood pressure, asthma, hypertension, and sleep apnea can be directly attributed to childhood obesity.
- Cardiovascular disease (CVD), diabetes and chronic kidney disease (CKD) account for approximately [a] quarter of the burden of disease in Australia, and just under two-thirds of all deaths. These three diseases often occur together and share risk factors, such as physical inactivity, overweight and obesity and high blood pressure." [15]

With heart disease being Australia's number one killer, and diabetes on the rise—affecting some 900,000 Australians—could sugar be to blame?

Studies have shown that sugar causes high blood pressure and cutting it out does reduce it. Lutsig believes sugar is addictive and makes us crave more. Personally, I believe this is the reason why most people cannot stop at one piece of chocolate. Food today is altered to trigger our sensory awareness. The result is that once we help ourselves to something, we can't stop. I confess I am a sugar addict; if I have a piece of cake or chocolate,

I find I will have to fight my craving for another sweet hit the rest of the day. If you think back to our ancestral days, it makes sense that eating fruit caused a craving for more fruit—therefore eating more and more—because it would have helped people eat enough in the summer and fall to fatten up and survive the harsh winter months.

This brings us to the debate on fructose versus glucose. Fructose is one type of sugar molecule and is what gives fruit its sweet flavour. And what is more natural to eat than fruit? Arguably, very little. But not all fructose is the same, and many people are confused about how much fruit to include in their diets. The short answer is that it varies based on the type of diet they consume.

Fructose ranks low on the glycemic index, which basically means it does not impact your blood glucose levels. That's a good thing. If people limited their consumption of fructose to just healthy fruits, your body would be able to process it with little effort. Unfortunately, canned and processed foods often add fructose to foods, and it comes in many forms, including high-fructose corn syrup, crystalline fructose, and agave. This type of fructose is processed in your liver, bypassing your gastrointestinal tract entirely. Your liver has to work hard to process it, and when consumed often enough, can even result in scarring. Fructose can also raise your triglycerides and increase your risk of heart disease.[16]

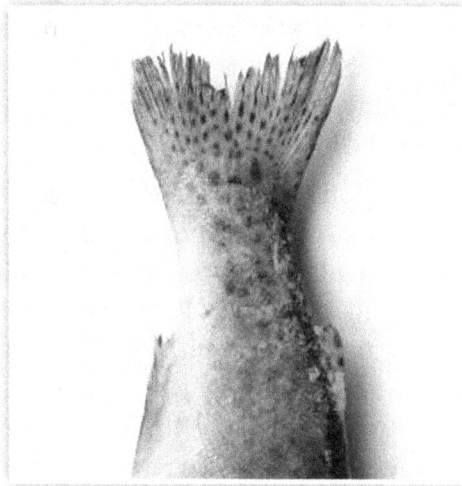

Glucose is another form of sugar but it is derived from starches. After consuming starches, your body converts them to glucose while raising blood sugar levels, as mentioned earlier. In an effort to stabilize the blood sugar, the body will prompt the pancreas to release the hormone insulin. It binds with the glucose and carries the molecules to the cells requiring extra energy, and stores anything leftover in the fat cells. If this eating pattern continues, eventually the pancreas becomes exhausted and is unable to efficiently release insulin any longer, leaving that person with chronically elevated blood glucose levels such as what is found in Type 2 diabetes or metabolic syndrome. Unfortunately, because insulin is now released in an inefficient manner, it is more difficult for the cells to get the insulin they need to 'unlock' the cell 'door' and allow nutrients inside, resulting in cell starvation.[16]

This is a problem that goes beyond body size as well; in other words, even if you are thin, this is an area to remain vigilant. It is possible to be lean and metabolically unhealthy. More than 40% of normal weight people show signs of metabolic disease. Visceral fat is the type of fat that is stored under the belly and around organs and this is where bigger health problems arise! It's the worst type of fat because it releases certain hormones that cause inflammation in various locations throughout the body. It concerns me how many children I see sucking down a Pop Top or Prima full of sugar and they have big bellies. It's not healthy nor is it 'cute puppy fat'—it's dangerous! It isn't fun when kids cry, but which is worse: hearing your children moan and whine because they can't have the chocolate Big M in their lunch order and an icy pole like the other kids, or you crying later when they are riddled with health issues? I'm not saying deprive them; instead, come up with creative options that are still healthy, such as fresh fruit kebabs or homemade icy poles so you can control the ingredients.

When in doubt, fresh fruit is a much better choice. Whole fruits contain only a small amount of fructose along with water, fibre, and other beneficial nutrients. When considering fruit choices, keep in mind which fruit is in season. Summer fruits tend to be higher in sugars. If you follow the raw food plan, feel free to consume large quantities of seasonal fruit; there is no reason to limit yourself. If you follow the RPP plan, fruit should be limited to two - three pieces per day. An even better option in winter is to select sprouts and grasses—they provide good energy with less sugar.

Refer to the reference below for more information.

Dietary Fats

Food For Health
TURNING THE FOOD PYRAMID ON ITS HEAD

Previously in this chapter I mentioned that the four types of fats are: saturated, trans, polyunsaturated, and monounsaturated. In general, dieticians and health experts recommend people reduce or eliminate saturated and trans fats from your diet.

However, coconut oil is an exception to the saturated fat rule. It is solid at room temperature like other saturated fats; however, it is a plant-based fat and offers many health benefits. *Organicfacts.net* states, "The health benefits of coconut oil include hair care, skin care, stress relief, cholesterol level maintenance, weight loss, boosted immune system, proper digestion and regulated metabolism. It also provides relief from kidney problems, heart diseases, high blood pressure, diabetes, HIV, and cancer, while helping to improve dental quality and bone strength. These benefits of oil can be attributed to the presence of lauric acid, capric acid and caprylic acid, and their respective properties, such as antimicrobial, antioxidant, anti-fungal, antibacterial and soothing qualities."[17]

One big diet myth to store in your brain is: consumed fat is not automatically stored as fat. All food is converted into energy to burn, and this includes fat. In fact, fat is useful for many of the functions required for a healthy body and helps you feel satiated when you consume it. You do not need to be afraid of fats, in fact, I recommend you eat good fats at every meal (avocado, nuts, seeds, etc).

Refer to the references below for more information.

REFERENCE	LOCATION
Dietary Fats	124

Vitamins and Minerals

When we make healthy food choices, our vitamin and mineral needs are usually met. However, if you are unaware of what your body needs from vitamins and minerals, it's hard to make a knowledgeable decision!

Fat-soluble vitamins are vitamins A, D, E, and K. They are found in fatty foods, such as oily fish, butter, and animal fats, and are important for many body processes. When you consume too much, excess fat-soluble vitamins are stored in the liver and fatty tissue until needed.[18]

Vitamin D remains a source of constant debate, as some medical authorities argue that the average person gets enough D from the sun. Our Paleolithic ancestors would certainly have received plenty of sun exposure during their daily lives, but in our current culture, many people today work indoors and may suffer from a lack vitamin D. Fatty ocean fish are a good source of vitamin D, but most other foods lack in it. If you don't get around 15 minutes of good sun exposure during the day, you may want to consider a good quality vitamin D supplement.

Water-soluble vitamins are vitamins C, all of the B vitamins, and folic acid and are found in vegies, fruits, and grains (although I do not recommend grains as a source). If you consume extra water-soluble vitamins, your body expels them in your urine.[18] Boiling or cooking these vitamins results in a loss of some nutrients, so raw or steaming are healthier options for your vegies and fruit.

Minerals are divided into macrominerals and trace minerals. Macro-minerals help your body convert food into energy, build strong teeth and bones, produce hormones, and control body fluids inside and outside your cells. They include calcium, magnesium, sodium, potassium, phosphorus, sulfur, and chloride and are found in meat, fish, fruit, vegetables, and nuts.[19]

Trace minerals are elements your body requires in very minute amounts. They include zinc, iron, iodine, manganese, copper, selenium, cobalt, and fluoride and are found in fish, meat, vegies, and nuts.[19] Zinc is the second largest trace element used by the body (second to iron) and is important for building your body's immune system, healing wounds, and digesting carbohydrates. Zinc is best sourced from animal proteins, so if you are following the raw food diet, supplementation is advised.

The best way to meet your vitamin and mineral requirements is to eat a diet with a wide variety of foods. To test for a zinc deficiency, buy zinc from a health store and swish around in your mouth. If the taste is mild or not present, you likely have a zinc deficiency. If so, review the reference below for supplementing in that area.

REFERENCE	LOCATION
Benefits of Zinc	128

Acid Vs. Alkaline

In 1931, German biochemist Dr. Otto Heinrich Warburg won the Nobel Peach Prize for his research on respiratory enzymes, or the impact of oxygen on the human body. His findings were astounding. It is unfortunate that his discovery is not better publicized, because it should be on the front page of every newspaper in the world.

1. Dr. Warburg discovered that the primary cause (meaning "present in all cases" of the disease) for the growth of cancer cells in the human body is lack of oxygen resulting in acidity.

2. All healthy cells require oxygen. If they lose access to oxygen for more than 48 hours, they can become cancerous, acidic cells.

3. Cancer cells *cannot* survive in the presence of oxygen.

4. Convert the cells to alkaline (above 7.365 pH) by carrying oxygen to the cells, and the cancer cells will starve.[20]

Cell oxygen is present in an alkaline state and the great news is that alkalinity in our bodies is something that we can control. In fact, Dr. Warburg was quoted in a speech to Nobel Laureates in German in 1966, stating, "It is indisputable that all cancer could be prevented if the respiration of body cells were kept intact."[20]

It is difficult to overstate how much this knowledge would change the world in terms of health if people were only aware of it. Regardless of the secondary causes of cancer—which are many—*we already know how to prevent it*. We simply need to work with our body to ensure our body's blood pH level stays alkaline, and that is done via organic green vegetables.

You can test your body's pH value using litmus paper. Take a strip, touch it to the inside of each of your cheeks and compare the colour with the chart provided. If highly acidic, purchase the urine dip stick and test via urine for better accuracy. Once you have your results, through proper nutrition you can ensure you maintain an optimal alkaline state.

Aside from the prevention of cancer, reducing acidity and maintaining alkalinity in the body is critical for overall health and the functioning of body processes. Happily, your body will naturally fight to maintain acidity, but if you consume increased levels of acid-based foods it has to deal with the acid, and there are consequences to it. For example, your body may "borrow" calcium from your bones when fighting to maintain your blood pH level, potentially leading to osteoporosis.[21] The stress of dealing with this health threat results in many problems, including "acne, eczema, osteoporosis, cancer, cardiovascular disease, premature aging, loss of hair, brittle nails, mental health problems, liver disease, kidney failure, psoriasis, fatigue, frequent coughs and colds, PMS, mood disorders, obesity, Type 2 diabetes, athletes foot, low sex drive, dizziness" and more.[21]

To reduce stress on your body and improve your health, learn which foods are higher or lower in acid content. Please consult the attachment in this section because awareness of the acid levels in foods is not simply intuitive. For example, fruits such as lemons, limes, and oranges contain acid but are processed as alkaline by the body; therefore, they have an alkaline affect upon the body. Fruit *juices*, however, are acidic.

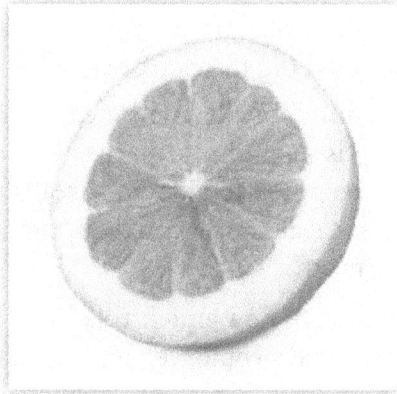

Interestingly, vinegars, while acidic by nature, have an alkaline effect upon the body and offer many health benefits. For example, apple cider vinegar can help balance your blood pH value rather than increase your acidity. I recommend supplementing your water with a slice of lemon in the morning, and a spoonful of diluted apple cider vinegar 30 minutes before your evening meal, to aid in easier food digestion throughout your day.

Refer to the references below for more information.

REFERENCE	LOCATION
Acid vs. Alkaline Foods	130
Green Vegies Article	http://www.food4health.com.au/green-vegetables/
Benefits of Apple Cider Vinegar	131

Danger of Overcooking

No doubt you've heard of the dangers of undercooking your food, due to the possible presence of certain types of bacteria. However, were you aware there is also additional health risks associated with overcooking your food?

When beef, fish, pork, and poultry are overcooked, chemicals such heterocyclic amines (HCAs) can form when high temperatures are applied to the meat. The more 'done' the meat, the more likely HCAs are present in the meat.[22]

In addition, the more food is overcooked, the more difficult it is for your body to digest it because the healthy nutrients in the food, such as the amino acids, are destroyed. Food should not be cooked beyond medium well, and using a meat thermometer is always recommended.

Danger of Microwaves

Microwaves have become so common in first world society it's often difficult to find a home without one. But just because they are found everywhere, are they actually safe? And is it okay to heat up your food in one?

To answer that question, consider Arielle Reynolds of Sussex. This ambitious student decided to conduct a microwave experiment for her school science project. She took filtered water, divided it into two equal parts, heated one half in the microwave, allowed it to cool, and watered two plants over the course of 9 days. The results showed that, over time, the microwaved water killed the plant. [23]

The obvious question is *why*?

Microwaves use non-ionizing radiation to warm up food by heating up the water particles in food, causing friction due to the heat, resulting in warm food. However, this friction heating alters the chemical structure in your food by converting the cells to carcinogens

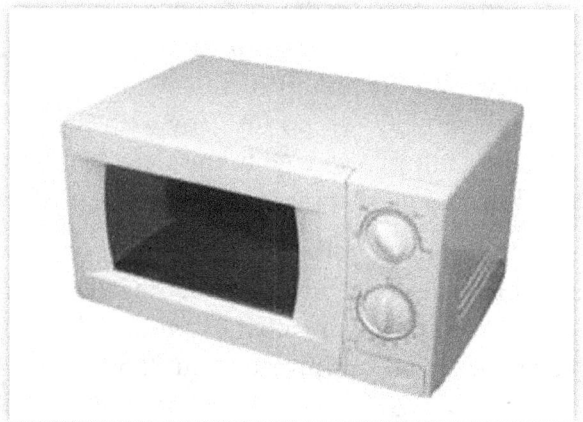

and toxins, and in the process, destroys the nutrients in the food that make it healthy to consume.

Consider the results of a Russian study that was published by the Atlantis Raising Educational Center in Portland, Oregon. While there was much to consider, a few highlights are below.

- "Microwaving prepared meats sufficiently to insure sanitary ingestion caused formation of d-Nitrosodienthanolamines, a well-known carcinogen.

- Microwaving milk and cereal grains converted some of their amino acids into carcinogens.

- Thawing frozen fruits converted their glucoside and galactoside containing fractions into carcinogenic substances.

- Extremely short exposure of raw, cooked or frozen vegetables converted their plant alkaloids into carcinogens.

- Carcinogenic free radicals were formed in microwaved plants, especially root vegetables."[24]

In addition, estimates go as high as *97% of the nutritional content of food* is lost in microwaving. The results were dire enough that the Soviet Union actually banned microwave ovens in 1976, and they stayed banned for over 20 years.[24]

Keep in mind also that while standards are high for microwave safety, they may not be high enough. Microwaves have been known to leak electromagnetic radiation if not sealed properly, especially as they begin to age through common wear and tear.[24]

Finally, consider the container used in your microwaving. It is important if using plastic that you confirm it is Bisphenol A (BPA) free to avoid toxins leaching into the food. When viewing the numbers on the bottom of any plastic container, do not use any with the numbers 3, 6, and 7 on them. For more information, go to the Care 2 Website at *www.care2.com*. Where possible, use glass containers instead of plastic for your food storage.

In summary, rather than assuming microwaves are a safe convenience for your household you are encouraged to do additional research on your own, including looking up the nine day plant experiment. You might decide you're better off warming up your family's meals via oven, light grilling, or other convectional heating method, where external heat is applied to the food rather than frictional heat. Your body will thank you!

○ TRUTHS ABOUT BREASTFEEDING

If you are a mum, or plan to be a mum in the future, this section is dedicated to you. There is a lot of controversy surrounding the benefits of breastfeeding, so please read the information in this section before making a decision against it.

Importance of Breastfeeding

You've heard it before—breastfeeding allows mum and baby to bond. But is it true or just coddling? Is it worth the soreness, the frustration, the constant pumping? What about the constant debate over where and when to breastfeed?

Consider the following list of breastfeeding benefits for your baby and decide for yourself.

- **It protects your baby from illness.** When you begin to produce milk you will initially produce colostrum that will contain secretory immunoglobulin A (IgA) which coats and protects your baby's mucosal membranes against germs. Your IgA is customized for your baby's health. If fact, if you get sick, your breast milk will produce the specific IgA needed to protect your baby from the illness. And the benefits of breastfeeding extend beyond infancy, even lowering your child's risk of developing childhood cancer and other chronic diseases later in life. [25]
- **It makes your baby smarter.** Breastfeeding is associated with increased cognitive development in babies due to the benefits of emotional bonding and the helpful fatty acids found in breast milk. [25]

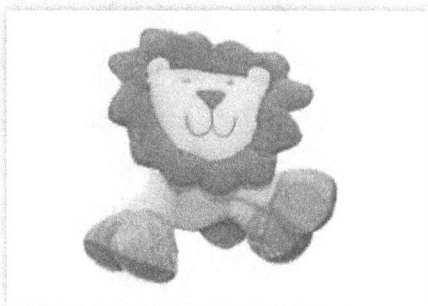

- **It helps prevent obesity.** Breastfeeding your baby can help your child develop appropriate hunger and satiety responses to food, developing a foundation for good eating skills that will influence them all their life. Also, breastfed babies have more leptin in their bodies—a hormone that is closely tied to monitoring appetite.[25]

In addition, breastfeeding is helpful to mum because it causes your body to release prolactin and oxytocin, hormones that cause you to feel relaxed and to experience a bonding love with your baby. Plus, the oxytocin also helps your body to heal more quickly after the experience of child birth[26] and lowers your risk of postpartum depression.[25]

Drawbacks of Formula

The alternative to breastfeeding is, of course, formula and these days, it is big business. Soy formula remains a popular alternative. And what about organic baby formula?

Again, take some time to review the potential problems with feeding your baby a diet of formula before making a decision.

- Studies have shown that babies offered cow or soy formula are more likely to develop allergies later.[25]
- As mentioned previously, soy mimics estrogen and causes hormone problems in women and men; this danger is exponentially increased in babies with developing bodies. "Critics say soy isoflavones are close enough to human estrogens to fool the body and cause early puberty in girls, promote breast cancer in women, reduce male fertility, cause thyroid dysfunction and delay or arrest the sexual maturation of boys."[27]
- Infant formulas are frequently processed under high heat which can trigger the formation of "advanced glycation end products (AGES)", which are "sugar molecules that can attach to and damage proteins" in a body. In addition, babies "switched from breast milk to commercial formula within the first year of life, their levels of AGEs doubled to levels found in people with diabetes" and had increased levels of insulin.[28]
- Even organic baby formula has issues; it has fewer pesticides but usually has brown rice syrup—which is known to have arsenic—

and few long-term studies have been conducted to determine
health impacts.[29]

- Cost! Breastfeeding is free while formula costs for a growing
  baby quickly add up.

Yes, there can be difficulties with breastfeeding. Sometimes it's not
particularly convenient or you may have to deal with a person who is less
than understanding. However, it is my hope the list above will give you
reason to consider breastfeeding as a blessing and useful option for feeding
your baby.

In a world of health problems, give your child the best fighting chance
they have at good health! It is truly a gift that will bless them throughout
their lives—and yours.

○ HANDLING CRITICISM

Before we close out Day 2, I owe you a word of warning. If you are a parent,
be prepared that once you choose a food plan and your family begins to
eat following your new food choices, you will begin to face criticism from
others. *Why can't your kids have some pizza? Don't you think your diet is a
little extreme? What will happen to your calcium levels if your don't drink
dairy?*

As a parent, you should be prepared to get comments and criticisms
about the food choices you are making for your family. By reading this book
you are arming yourself with knowledge—which is a great start.

However, don't be afraid to express the truth. Try the following
responses when you are faced with curious questions from others.

Q. What do you mean you don't eat bread?!

A. That's right; I don't eat bread or any grains as it affects my body and
I get bloated.

Q. Why you don't give you child sandwiches?

A. They react badly to grain as well—most people do. It's just easier if
we all cut it out.

Q. You don't consume dairy? Where do you get your calcium?

A. Believe it or not, you can't absorb the calcium from dairy. Plus, certain food combinations (for example, milk and cereal) prevent you from absorbing it anyway. Now they are proving too much calcium is linked to osteoporosis. I believe we get all we need from fruits and vegetables.

Q. It's important to eat grains. Where do your kids get their fibre?

A. Cereals and processed foods don't agree with me, and the sugar content is through the roof. Most of the package is simply false advertising. I've even seen a cereal advertised as containing protein—it was nothing more than powdered whey, which is not healthy! Fibre is better sourced from fruits and greens.

Q. Your kids' brain development will slow down if you don't eat carbohydrates!

A. I eat carbs, potatoes, sweet potatoes, and other starchy vegetables. I would never deprive my family.

Q. Can you eat gluten free products?

A. I can; I just chose to limit the amount of them as they often contain other unhealthy ingredients.

Q. It's fine to let them have a few lollies here and there. They're kids—it's a treat!

A. I agree. If my kids are invited to a party I'm not going to keep them from going. However, I like to educate my kids and prevent the sugar high if possible. They know what's in a lot of birthday party food and how bad it is for health. I'm proud because I'm giving them the information we didn't have when we were kids, and then I can let them make the decision. Quite often my daughter will opt for an apple than a lollie believe it or not!

Q. What *do* you eat?

A. I'm a big fan of food! I eat a lot of fresh fruit and vegies. Since changing my diet, I've been able to get really creative in the kitchen with my meals. I really enjoy getting my hands 'dirty', so to speak.

○ TRANSITIONING TO NEW DIETARY CHOICES

You have a lot of changes in front of you—for you and your family. Change is never easy. First, know that it's fine to start slowly by making gradual changes so that people are not quite so shocked and confused by your lifestyle changes, and your kids have time to adapt.

If you are concerned about jumping into all the food changes at once, consider making the changes gradually by utilizing the following schedule:

- Month 1—Update your pantry
- Month 2—Eliminate dairy
- Month 3—Remove all grain
- Month 4—Eliminate sugar

As you go through these changes, always be prepared for hungry kids (and you!) by keeping a fresh fruit and a vegie platter in the fridge. Slice carrots, celery, capsicum, sprouts and more so that hungry people have a quick healthy option. The more they nibble from it, the more their taste buds will transition to healthy, clean eating. Break the biscuit habit!

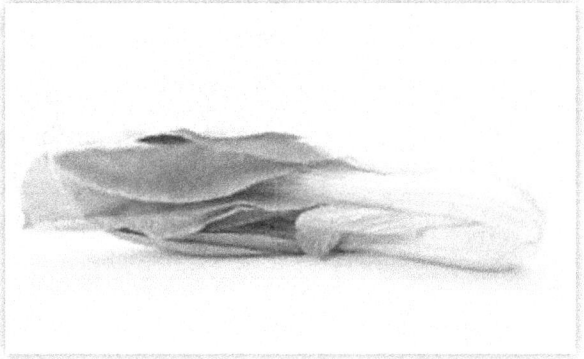

> **TIP:** *You know you are eating healthy when your fridge is near empty except for fresh produce!*

Another option to ease the transition is to simply try 'swapping out' one food choice on your plate for another, better food choice. Below is a list of suggested 'food swaps' that offer you better nutritional value than their replacements.

CURRENT FOOD CHOICE	BETTER FOOD CHOICES
Bread	Nori sheets / Lettuce / Kale
Store bought snacks	Buy a dehydrator and make your own dried fruit, fruit roll-ups, jerky, crackers, and chips
Grains	Quinoa, oats, and rice (occasionally)
Rice	Cauliflower rice or parsnip rice (recipes in Appendix B)
Milk	Nut milks, coconut milk, rice milk, coconut yogurt (recipes in Appendix B)
Seeds	Chia seeds
Ice cream	Blend frozen fruits (banana and fresh dates are my fave!)
Desserts	A quick internet search will pull up many recipes that are grain, dairy, and sugar free!

If you are transitioning from a diet including meat to the raw foods plan, you can also do a slower transition for that as well. Start by adding a vegan source of protein to your meals 2 to 3 times a weeks, and limit the amount of red meat you consume. Gradually increase the number of days per week until you reach your goal.

TIP: *By adding just two vegan meals a week into your home, not only will you be healthier for choosing more alkaline sources for protein, but you are also helping to fight poverty and world famine—it takes a lot of grain to feed one animal!*

○ TAKE ACTION

Day 2 has a wealth of information for you to read and consider about your health, but simply reading words on a page will not change your life. Act on the commitments you made above by choosing action steps from the list below to start today!

Step 1. Choose one of the suggested food plans: raw foods or RPP (Raw Plus Protein).

Step 2. Print the applicable grocery reference sheets and place them in a binder with section dividers.

Step 3. Label the **second** divider "Food Cheat Sheets".

This binder is going to be used to get your life organized. Label it "Mum's Organizer" or whatever you like! As you read through this book, you will get instructions to continue to add sheets to your binder. It should prove to be a useful reference and organization tool that will help you in forming good habits.

DAY 3:
Sustainability

3

"*Sustainability is a new idea to many people, and many find it hard to understand. But all over the world there are people who have entered into the exercise of imagining and bringing into being a sustainable world. They see it as a world to move toward not reluctantly, but joyfully, not with a sense of sacrifice, but a sense of adventure. A sustainable world could be very much better than the one we live in today.*"

~ Donella H. Meadows, ~
~ The Limits to Growth: The 30-Year Update ~

HOW IS YOUR NEW nutritional plan going? Hopefully you are making little changes each day to incorporate those good, healthy foods you have chosen.

For Day 3 we are going to address sustainable living—what it is, as well as some practical steps on how to incorporate sustainable living into your lifestyle.

O **SUSTAINABILITY CONCEPT**

There are a lot of definitions floating around about sustainability, but the essence of it is to limit the amount of wastage in your life by reducing your resources and choosing to live a simpler lifestyle. This varies from something as modest as recycling to the extreme of installing toilets in your house that turn human waste into compost.

Aside from personal choice, where you live and what you do will offer limitations on how much of a sustainable lifestyle you can practically manage or incorporate. For example, no doubt your local council likely already organizes recycling in your neighborhood, but your Body Corporate may not allow you to have a chicken coop in your backyard in a suburb.

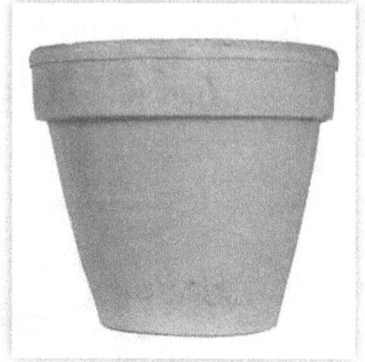

The topics included below will be simple and easy to apply for almost any but the most challenging home-based living situations and all of them will focus on areas that can improve the quality and cost of your food resources.

○ LIVING SUSTAINABLY

Maybe you are wondering why sustainability is important. I've included it in this book for a few basic reasons, but to sum them all up in a single phrase: sustainable living benefits *you*. It offers you cost savings and healthier living options, so even if this is not a lifestyle choice you have considered before, please read on to discover how easy it is to live with a lighter carbon footprint (and a smaller waistline).

Identify Habits of Wastage

Most of us say we want to be more environmentally friendly, don't we? Now is the time to talk the talk and walk the walk. To do that, print "How Sustainable Are You?" and fill it out.

REFERENCE	LOCATION
How Sustainable Are You?	133

This worksheet will help you evaluate how much effort you have put into living sustainably.

To remind you of our goals, this evaluation is not intended to be self-condemning, but rather to encourage honest reflection, and to perhaps consider areas where you think you could change. Sustainability is not a requirement—just a good idea that benefits you!

Reject Bad Habits

Are you surprised at how sustainable you are-—or do you have room for improvement? Are you willing to admit that you've had some bad habits and turn a corner in your life? Or will you continue to put off change for 'one more day'?

Procrastination is easy to settle into. It's convenient, it's easy—and it's a cop out. You will *not* be a 'terrible person' if you do not take a little extra initiative to change your life in this area today, but it is a missed opportunity. How many of us are familiar with the concept of "I'll eat better tomorrow", and tomorrow never comes? This bad habit applies to every area of our lives that could stand a little improvement. Don't wait. When the door opens, walk through it!

Choose Sustainability

If you find you could do a little better, no worries. Most people find they can and want to do more. If you have room to grow in this area, make a choice to do just one baby step better, and you will have made a difference. No regrets here—just jump in where you are and get started! Which brings us to your commitment...

Commitment #3: **Choose one new sustainability activity and start it within one week.**

○ WHAT CAN I DO TO LIVE MORE SUSTAINABLY?

No doubt, you already recycle. Australian laws and availability for recycling make it simple and easy to do, so if you are not recycling, please make a decision to start. The efforts of one multiplied by the efforts of many have a huge impact in reducing the amount of rubbish in the tip.

However, there are more options that are simple and easy to do. Let's talk about a few more ways you can live a 'cleaner' lifestyle.

Food For Health
TURNING THE FOOD PYRAMID ON ITS HEAD

Planting a Garden

Planting a garden is one of the easiest ways to live a sustainable lifestyle. If offers you cost savings, because you eat the fruit (and herbs and vegies) of your labors, and it offers you exercise and fresh air (vitamin D). It requires some effort to get started, but after that, a relatively small amount of effort will keep it going.

Building raised planter boxes is as simple as nailing together four pieces of wide, untreated timber (do NOT use pressure treated timber as it has poisons in it) at the corners. Put the box in place where you want it, line the bottom with a small layer of sand or small rocks for better drainage, and fill with good quality dirt. Voila! Insert plants and enjoy. If you are not inclined to build your own, any nursery sells planter boxes you can use. Large terracotta pots are also a good choice.

Below are some tips for getting started on your first garden.

1. **Plant a variety of colour in your fruit and vegetables**, because the pigments indicate the nutrients available in the plant. The wider the colour variety on your plate, the more nutrients you are absorbing.

2. **Choose the number of plants carefully**, since some plants continue to produce throughout the season, such as capsicum and tomatoes, while others produce only once and must be replanted, such as carrots and corn.

3. **For the lowest initial time investment**, try to choose plants that continue to produce throughout the season—you can add the others later when you are a gardening veteran.

4. **Grow a garden of herbs first** if the thought of planting vegies or fruits is intimidating to you. It will build your confidence level. You will see how hardy plants can really be and you will want to expand your garden later.

5. **Go organic.** Refuse to use synthetic fertilizers and pesticides, and you will know that all of the produce in your garden is the cheapest option for organic produce that money can buy!

6. **Composting is easy.** Anytime you have vegetable scraps, grass clippings, fruit rinds, and more—throw them into your garden! Cover with a bit of dirt and forget about it. Within six months

you will be amazed at how healthy, lush, and fertile your soil is, and all with only minimal effort.

7. **Choose native plants.** By doing this, you increase your chances of a generous crop and reduce the amount of time spent fighting insects or illness.[30]

Start with a small box and work your way into a big beautiful garden. No doubt it will not be long before you begin to view your living art with pride! It feels good to the soul to be able to grow your own food and provide for yourself, and the benefits far outweigh the small time commitment required to maintain it.

Obviously a critical factor in planting your new garden is the time of year! Australia is a mix of climates and it's important to consider where you live when determining when to plant and what to plant in your garden.

The good news is that there is an easy resource to consult no matter what time of year it is when you get your garden ready to plant.

- Go to http://www.abc.net.au/gardening/vegieguide/
- Select the climate you live in on the map
- Select the current month at the top of the page

A list of current plants in their growing season will be available to scroll through. Click on the plants you are interested in to learn more information. It's that easy!

Fermented Plants

The benefits of fermented foods were covered earlier, so jump back to Day 2 if you need a reminder. This section is to discuss how you can easily and inexpensively add more fermented foods into your diet by making your own. You want these healthy microbes in your body to help you digest all the food you eat!

To ferment your own vegies you will need clean, sterilized mason jars and good quality organic vegies, including celery. With those ingredients, you can add other vegies to the mix and make whatever fermented vegies you prefer. Make several jars at once and your 'crop' of fermented vegetables will last you for weeks—making mealtime even more convenient!

Reference the attachment "Fermenting Your Vegies" for a few simple steps on how to safely and effectively ferment your own vegetables.

Here are a few extra tips:

- Peel the skins off of vegies before fermenting to avoid bitterness.
- Add small amounts of fresh organic ginger, garlic, onion, or herbs for flavour but only in small amounts—a little goes a very long way!
- Add salt! Salt offers many benefits to the fermenting process by:
  - Enhancing flavor
  - Making the vegies crunchier
  - Preventing mushy vegies
  - Inhibits the growth of any harmful bacteria [31]
- Using whey as a starter culture will result in mushier vegies, so keep texture in mind when you ferment.
- The starter culture you choose will also affect the flavor, so if you don't like one batch, try a different one next time! Options include celery brine, salt, whey, kefir, using juice from a previous fermented batch, and commercially produced cultures.

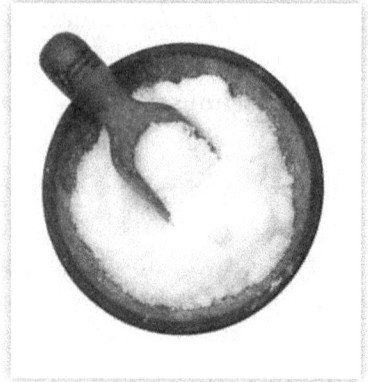

In addition to making fermented vegies, another great fermenting option is making your own kombucha! People that love sugary, carbonated drinks or cordial will find kombucha a healthier and delicious alternative! It's basically like brewing tea but with a starter 'mushroom' or 'pancake' (or starter culture) and a few extra ingredients. Compared to the $4 bottles you buy at the store, you can make your own for much cheaper.

Any recipe for kombucha includes sugar, but don't panic! The sugar is food for your kombucha mushroom (or SCOBY) and is what creates the probiotics and acids that make kombucha so healthy! It has far less sugar than regular soda and it serves a required purpose, so don't be tempted to reduce the sugar amount in the recipe for that reason.

Check out the references below for more information.

REFERENCE	LOCATION
Fermenting Your Vegies	134
Making Kombucha	134

Sprouts

If you want a good boost of enzymes, vitamins, minerals, antioxidants, and trace minerals, than sprouted foods are a good addition to your diet. Being low calorie and low in fat means they are also a flexible and easy addition to any meal—plus they have around 20% - 35% protein content.

Sprouting increases the nutritional value in a seed by increasing the vitamin A, B, and C content. They are simple to start, easy to grow, and have been consumed for over 5000 years. That's quite a history! And considering that a mere few ounces of seeds produces over a pound of sprouts, you will get good benefits for your small investment.

Any seed, bean, grain, or nut can be sprouted although I recommend choosing organic as the safest, healthiest seeding option.

Every now and then a case of salmonella poisoning (associated with sprouts) is announced in the news, so perhaps you might be wondering if sprouting is truly safe? Let me put your mind at ease. Safety issues are only a concern with regards to how the seeds are handled—commercially grown seeds are usually treated with pesticides and chemicals, and are not handled with care. Per the website Health Eating Advisor, "Organic seeds have never been implicated in a single case of salmonella poisoning." Stay organic and you have no worries![32]

Read "Easy Steps to Sprouting" for simple steps to growing your own fresh, delicious, sprouts!

REFERENCE	LOCATION
Easy Steps to Sprouting	138

Composting

Compost is the natural process of decomposing organic material, or for a more practical definition, lush, healthy dirt that is chock full of nutrients.

As plants grow they deplete the nutrients in the soil they grow in, so it is important to replenish those nutrients by adding healthy organic material.

For established beds, occasionally adding leftover vegie and fruit cuttings from your kitchen—as well as grass, leaves, sticks, etc.—straight onto the soil (cover food with soil) will help replenish those nutrients. However, you may want to add new footage to your landscaping or build another raised plant bed, and in those cases, having a stockpile of compost available when you need it is both a money saver and time saver. Plus, compost is good for rebuilding soil that is overly clay or sandy, transforming it into loamy soil—so rather than making a whole new bed from fresh compost, you can mix your current soil with compost for better texture and nutrients, and save yourself some money.

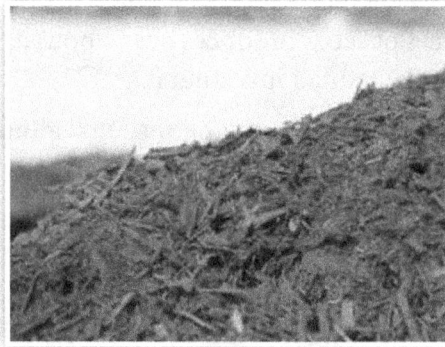

Creating compost can be simple or complicated, cheap or expensive. You're probably a busy responsible adult, so we'll assume simple is best here. If you want complicated or expensive, you can buy fancy, pricey barrels that will allow you to easily turn your compost. Turning your compost on a regular basis will increase the speed of decomposition, but it isn't a requirement, so if going the cheapest route is your preference, all you need is a stainless steel metal or non-toxic plastic barrel with a lid.

To start your compost pile:

- Find a suitable bin. Size is up to you, as is mobility. You can find a purpose-made bin, but typically they will be more expensive. Whatever you choose, it should be made of stainless steel (to prevent rust) or a non-toxic plastic that will stand up to the sun, and ideally, it should have a removable lid.

- Begin collecting organic matter: food scraps, leaves, branches, grass clippings, etc.
- Toss all of the organic matter into the bin. Add a little water to increase the humidity and decomposition rate, close the lid, and leave it somewhere where the container is exposed to sunlight.
- Periodically stir the contents or roll your container, and continue to add scraps and clippings on a regular basis. When it gets dry, add a little water again.
- Whenever you need good compost, take what you need from the bin and leave the rest. It is literally a renewable resource!

Great organic items for your bin:

- kitchen scraps and coffee grounds
- manure from horses, cows, and rabbits
- green grass, weed, and shrub clippings, as well as dried clippings of any kind
- branches (be aware these will take longer to decompose if they are not shredded first)

Avoid throwing these items into the bin:

- newspapers or other printed materials (the ink and/or paper can be poisonous or toxic)
- timber that has been pressure treated for outdoor use
- meat or animal fat (the scent will attract animals)
- ashes
- manure from dogs or cats[33]

While you really cannot mess up the composting process, the one caution is to be sure you are not ONLY putting in kitchen scraps in your bin. Putting in grass clippings and other heavy fibrous materials ensures that you don't have a steaming hot pile of rubbish in your yard. As long as you are putting in your yard clippings every now and then, you should be fine. If your compost bin ever starts to smell, increase the grass clippings and reduce the food waste.

Composting is one of the easiest things you will ever do, and saves the cost of buying those expensive bags of dirt from the store—plus, "homemade" compost is as good as anything you can buy! It's also a bonus that you can feel good about protecting the environment by using natural products on your plants and reducing the amount of waste that might go into a landfill. The wildlife will love you for it!

○ TAKE ACTION

Day 3 has a lot of practical application in it, and they are life changes that involve getting up and active! While I encourage you to implement *every one* of these simple, sustainability options at some point, unless you are retired or not working, it probably isn't realistic to start everything at once. Instead pick one, and act on it.

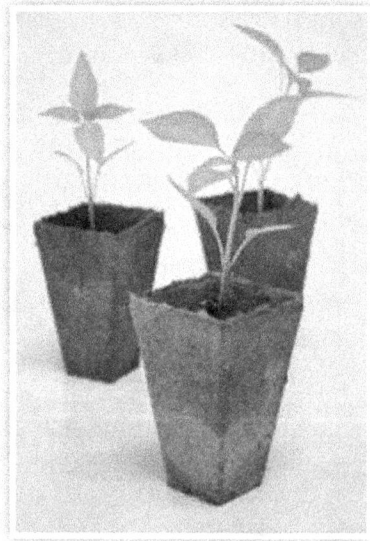

Step 1. Pick one new sustainability activity to work into your home life this week: start a garden, ferment vegies, grow your own sprouts, or build your own compost pile.

Step 2. Print the applicable reference sheets from this section for your organizer you started on Day 2.

Step 3. Label the third divider "Sustainability Cheat Sheets" and insert your newly printed sheets there.

Once you have taken action, Day 3 is done. Now on to Day 4!

DAY 4:
House Cleaning

4

> "I hate housework. You make the beds, you wash the dishes, and six months later you have to start all over again."

~ **Rivers** ~

BY NOW YOU SHOULD have chosen a meal plan and something new to make your carbon footprint on this planet a little smaller. You are making progress—you are improving your life while others only talk about it!

But what about that *elusive* lifestyle status symbol of—a clean home? Is a clean, well-organized home even a possibility anymore?

We live in a society where we work hard and play harder. As a good work/life balance becomes more and more difficult to achieve without adding to our stress levels, it might be tempting to throw a clean house to the wind. Who has time? Add kids to the mix and it seems like failure is guaranteed. When it comes to choosing between making dinner for the kids and dusting, it's easy to see which option will win.

Welcome to a better option!

Challenges of a Clean Home

The biggest obstacle we have to overcome for a clean, happy, functioning home is ourselves. Perhaps you are thinking, "*I already know this—the kids leave a trail behind them from the door to their bedroom, so no shocker there.*"

But that isn't what I mean.

As people, and especially mums, we tend to view cleaning as all or nothing. We don't view ten minutes as a valuable chunk of time to do anything, and if the house isn't perfect, then we just won't bother putting up much of a fight (until family invites themselves over, of course). However this type of thinking can be self-destructive.

Once again, how we clean our home—the approach and mindset we take—probably comes from our parents, and likely our mums. However, many of our mums lived at home. It was a different time with different goals and family expectations.

Please take this to heart: if you work outside the home, and you try to match what your mum did in 12 hour days all within your 4 evening hours after work (or whatever is applicable to your schedule), *you will drive yourself mad*. Give up on the mentality that it's even possible. It's an unhealthy expectation—throw it away.

However, you should also beware the danger of perfection. You don't need a home where you eat off of the floor; you need a safe, happy, and comfortable environment for your family. Please do not stress yourself over the fantasy image that a sterilized home is the ideal.

Most people fall into one of two opposite categories: they clean non-stop and they are miserable from the stress, or they have largely given up and are burdened with the stress of living in a dirty home.

Happiness, dear friends, is found in the middle.

Identify Bad Housecleaning Habits

Are you curious about how your personal housecleaning habits stack up? Fill out the "What Are My Housecleaning Habits?" worksheet and find out!

REFERENCE	LOCATION
What Are My Housecleaning Habits?	140

This worksheet will help you evaluate how much time and effort you put into cleaning, as well as the results of your effort, big or small. Take a few minutes now to fill it out—and be honest!

Reject Bad Housecleaning Habits

It is key for you to understand that bad habits are what got you into your current situation. It was a lack of routine and self-discipline; no plan and the wrong level of effort. And because this happened over time, it will be corrected over time. This requires a change of heart. When you follow the routines below, just view each task in front of you as something to complete and *don't worry about anything else.* Take each task one at a time. You will not accomplish it all at once, so refuse to feel pressure to do so.

However, there is also no need to give up entirely and leave the house full of clutter and crumbs. You can do this! You just need the right mindset and tools to complete the task.

Choose Good Housecleaning Habits

All house cleaning activities can be split into two major activities. No matter what you are doing in your house, it involves one of these two components:

- Cleaning
- De-cluttering/organizing

Sometimes when people say they don't like to clean, what they really mean is that they don't like to put clutter away. Other times, they mean they don't like to scrub something. And every single one of us has something about cleaning or organizing that we don't like to do. There are typically certain tasks or rooms in the house that people hate to clean. In general, the list usually looks something like this, from most disliked to least:

- bathrooms
- kitchen
- laundry
- bedrooms
- common living spaces

Here are the new and entirely appropriate rules for a clean home today. Repeat these three points until you know they are true. In fact, print this page, cut out this list, and stick it to your mirror.

> **My new focus for cleaning my home:**
>
> *1. I accept I will not have a clean house overnight.*
>
> *2. I understand the key to a clean house is following simple daily routines.*
>
> *3. I believe I will eventually have a sparkling clean home by cleaning only 30 minutes a day, and I am okay with that.*

The most important thing about having a clean living space is to build good routines, and good routines are built on good habits. Therefore, the solution to a clean home is to build good habits. Pay attention because this is critical: *it is more important to build the habits than it is to try to clean up the house in a weekend and then try to 'maintain' it.* The routines are the foundation and require 'practice'. If you try to skip that step—clean up the whole house and believe you can maintain your flurry of effort by suddenly implementing the daily routines—you will find you did not develop the habits necessary to maintain the cleanliness, and your house will slowly sink back into a disaster zone. There is no shortcut. The 'long way'—the less stressful way—is the right way. This ties to the next commitment.

Commitment #4: **Choose to create and maintain a clean household by implementing 30 minute daily routines.**

Do not clean or de-clutter your kid's rooms. If they are big enough to have their own room and make a mess with clutter, they are big enough to learn the basics of cleaning that mess. You will help them to learn their own routines, and when mum is cleaning, they will clean too. *Kids love using timers.* Help them the first few times and after that, they will clean when you do, and then you will inspect their room. You will be teaching them good habits they will use the rest of their lives, so do not underestimate the importance of this gift. Kids do not learn to clean by watching you—they learn by doing.

We are going to harness the power of your 30 minutes per day to get your house in order *over time.* To do that we're going to work smarter and not harder, and it will involve a little preparation. The first thing you're going to do is put together your Clean-Up Caddy.

Building Your Clean-Up Caddy

Buy a cheap, simple plastic carry-all with a handle--something deep enough to hold cleaning items. Even a decent sized bucket with a handle will work. Inside your Clean-up Caddy you will need the following items:

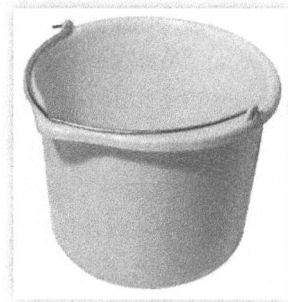

- Timer
- Gloves
- Quality microfiber cloths
- Scrubber brush or coarse sponge
- Spray bottle with vinegar and water mix (recipe in Appendix A)
- Spray bottle with toilet cleaner (recipe in Appendix A)
- Container of Scrubbing Cleaner (recipe in Appendix A)
- Mix Household Surface Grime Cleaner, when needed (recipe in Appendix A)
- Extra baking soda

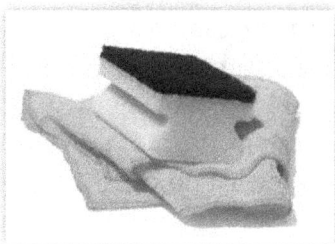

Think of this little collection of tools as a force to accomplish your task. The kids should also get their own cleaning tools, safe and appropriate for their age.

- The Kid Clean-Up Caddy should have the following items:
- Bucket
- Timer (or you can work together off your timer)
- Clean rags or paper towels
- Spray bottle with vinegar and water (or water only), if age appropriate

Cleaning Routine

Now that you have your Clean-Up Caddies ready to go, it's time to start cleaning!

Food For Health

The routines are split by day of the week. Read through them in advance now, and make minor adjustments to suit your lifestyle. However, do NOT change the following rules:

- Never continue cleaning in the same spot after the timer has buzzed. *Respect your time.*
- Once your routines are established, believe in them and use them faithfully.

REFERENCE	LOCATION
Monday - Friday Cleaning Routine	142
Saturday Cleaning Routine	145
Sunday Cleaning Routine	147
6 Month Deep Cleaning Routine	149
Household Cleaning Recipes	152

Start with the Monday - Friday list, and add the weekend list as soon as possible.

Every 6 months you will need to do some deeper cleaning around the house. For this type of cleaning, you will want to reserve a weekend or two. Since this is more strenuous, tedious cleaning, go slower and take a 10 - 15 minute break every hour (use your timer)! If you push yourself too hard and don't rest or get proper fluids, you will wear yourself down faster, get sore, and you won't want to do it again in 6 months.

As you work on your routine you will find that it will take you less and less time to complete your cleaning in the main areas where you clean daily. Move quickly and even if the bathroom vanity looks clean, still give it a quick swipe so that it *stays clean.* You will also find that many times the kids will start to respect how clean the house is and do their part to reduce their mess as well. As you get faster and cleaning needs decrease, you can use that extra time for yourself, or if you want, you can pick a bonus activity from the list on Sunday to complete.

However, the biggest thing to work on is your heart! Stop viewing housework as a chore to endure. No doubt you developed that viewpoint over time because it frustrated you. Most people do not love the action of cleaning, but they do love the feel of a beautiful, clean, comfortable home.

Get there through baby steps and you won't have the negative feelings to deal with anymore.

Take Action

Day 4 addresses something that can be difficult for any busy family to manage. It may be a while before you have a home that looks like one in the commercials, but that's okay—you can still have a home that you are proud of and you won't mind if family or friends drop in unexpectedly!

Step 1. Put together the clean-up caddies.

Step 2. Print the housecleaning lists for your organizer .

Step 3. Label the fourth divider "Housecleaning Lists" and insert your newly printed sheets behind it.

Once you have completed the steps above and your first day of clean-up routines, you can move on to Day 5!

DAY 5:
Healthy Lifestyle

"To laugh often and much; to win the respect of intelligent people and the affection of children; to earn the appreciation of honest critics and to endure the betrayal of false friends.

To appreciate beauty; to find the best in others; to leave the world a bit better whether by a healthy child, a garden patch, or a redeemed social condition; to know that even one life has breathed easier because you have lived. This is to have succeeded."

~ Ralph Waldo Emerson ~

YOU'VE MADE IT TO Day 5! And today is a very exciting day because it focuses on a complete picture of your health and ensures you are taking care of *you*.

Perhaps you are thinking, *but I'm already working on my nutrition*? And that's fantastic! But your health is more than just feeding your body. A truly healthy lifestyle includes proper attention to your physical body, as well as your mental and emotional health, your relationships with others, and living a full-bodied life that is rich in experiences.

The interesting thing about the concept of 'taking care of yourself' is that most people know this to be true, yet very few do it. We all *say* that we should take care of ourselves. In fact, many of us are quick to advise our friends they should take care of themselves, but when it comes to our own life, we fail to act. There is a stark contrast between what we say we believe and our actions, and we really have to bridge that gap because this is an important issue.

○ CHALLENGES OF LIVING A HEALTHY LIFESTYLE

Taking care of *you* is important. If you have a family or pets, they rely on you to be around for help and encouragement. That means you have to make sure you take care of yourself so that you can be there for them! A worn out, tired, frustrated person cannot encourage or support anybody in any way that is really significant. Do you want to be there for your kids? Your significant other? Your parents? Other family and friends? Then a balanced amount of time must be spent nourishing your soul as well as your body.

Don't take these elements of your life for granted—they impact every facet of your life, from your mental health to your ability to deal with stress and big life events. The only difference between a life thin on experience and joy, and a life packed with memories is the decision to live that life! Money is not a factor here. It expands your choices, but does not limit your ability, so read on for tips on taking care of every facet of you!

Identify Unhealthy Lifestyle Habits

Before jumping into ideas and tips for living that well-rounded life we all imagine in our deepest thoughts, take a few minutes to examine what you do now.

REFERENCE	LOCATION
Identify Your Unhealthy Lifestyle Habits	155

This worksheet will help you evaluate how much time and effort you invest in yourself. Are you spending any time on you? Are you nurturing those important relationships in your life? Time for a little honest self-evaluation!

Reject Unhealthy Lifestyle Habits

Once you have completed your worksheet, score it. What was your score?

- Which section did you score the strongest? (Congrats!)
- Which section could you improve on? (No worries! Start today!)

Food For Health

This list requires some extra evaluation than in the previous chapters, because these activities require tapping into a resource which is strictly limited in quantity—time. All of the items on that list require time, and we only have 24 hours in a day.

In case you are concerned, in no way am I suggesting that you should be checking 'daily' on all of those items—not only would that not be possible, but you would go mental even attempting it! However, to make time for the things in life that are *truly* important, we need to have an intentional purpose to include the important things. You might need to examine where you are devoting your time and see if you can make some adjustments to ensure you are living a balanced, healthy lifestyle that nurtures yourself and your relationships with family and friends.

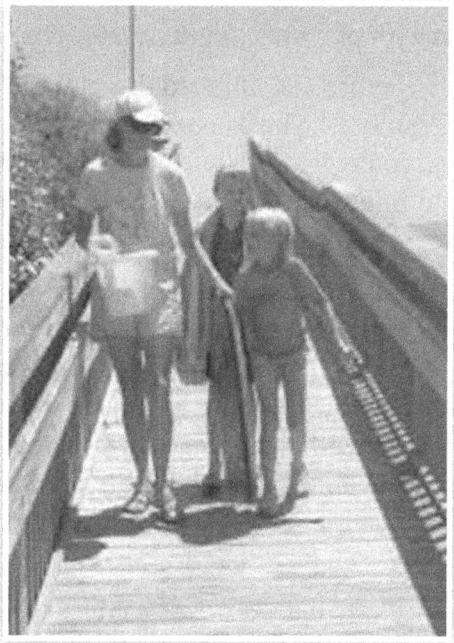

Do you have any negative habits that are bad for your health or time wasters? You know what activities are bad for you—smoking, excessive drinking, video game obsession, reading books for two hours a night, etc. Sometimes it's as simple as watching TV or movies for a couple hours (or longer) each evening. Many of these things can be okay for you in moderation, but they can be carried too far. In fact, as mums, sometimes we can get burned out because we don't take care of ourselves, and then we eventually look for an escape. We gain a hobby but unintentionally turn it into an obsession.

Honestly examine where you are with your life and where you want to be. Is there something you can cut away? Then do it. If it isn't contributing to the well-being of you, your partner, your kids, or friends and family, it's *hurting* you because it is *stealing time away that could be spent with them*. Get rid of the time wasters.

It's important to relax every day. Time is just like money in this aspect—we only get so much of it. It comes in limited quantities. Therefore, make sure you *invest* your time in the right areas.

Choose Healthy Lifestyle Habits

As with previous chapters, let's start small and build big!

Perhaps as you read through the section on "rejection" you now feel a bit guilty. Maybe you have some bad habits in your life you are not proud of and you've had to confront them. Moments of self-examination of the heart and mind, our actions—they can be tough. However, it's the people who refuse to consider where they could make changes that lack joy in their lives.

Guilt helps you realize where you might be making a mistake, but once you've realized it, make a fresh decision to change and take action right then. Do it. Do it right now. Before you even read past this paragraph, if there is a particular area where you feel some conviction, tell your lover you love them, spend 5 minutes with your kids, call your mum—whatever it is, just do it. Then come back to this and keep reading, and know you've already made a difference! I promise you, the guilt will melt away. You can change. Things can be different!

Now that you've considered the possibility that changes could be in order, let's talk about priorities. Priority does not mean the order of spending time with people, but rather, when circumstances force you to choose between two activities, you use the priority list to help you make your decision.

Your priority list:

- You
- Spouse/Partner
- Kids
- Friends/Parents/Extended Family
- Community Activities

Every day, the most important people in your life should get 15 minutes of quality time with you.

- First there is you—that is 15 minutes spent on yourself.

- If you have a partner, there should be another 15 minutes spent with him or her (alone).
- If you have kids, invest another 15 minutes spent with each child.

Before you start to feel panicky about this time investment, please read the context of how these recommendations should be applied.

- The timeframe is your goal, not the law. *Quality is more important than quantity.* Fifteen minutes of distracted conversation is not fulfilling the spirit of this concept. If it turns out you're extra busy and you can only give the kids 5 minutes each, just make it the best quality 5 minutes you can.
- This time can be spread out over the course of the day. For example, you may get up early (before the family wakes up) and spend 5 minutes meditating, and then in the evening, you may take a 10 minute bubble bath. Time spent with the kids may be 10 minutes helping with homework, and 5 minutes tucking them in at night.
- If your time is completely maxed out (this should be rare!) to the point that you get home late and you don't have the time to spend with everybody, time with your partner is a higher priority than time with the kids (more on this later).

Now that you have a better understanding of proper healthy lifestyle choices, commit to pursuing it.

Commitment 5: **Choose to take care of your overall physical, mental, and emotional health and to nurture healthy relationships in your life.**

Apply these changes gradually. Start with applying 1 week of YOU time (or longer if you feel stressed about it) before trying the others. Get your YOU time squared away first. Then the next week add time with your partner, and so on down the priority list.

○ NOURISHING YOU

The first habit you need to develop is time for you, and to make this a little more significant, think of it as an acronym: YOU = Your Opportunity to

Unwind. The focus of YOU time is more than physical relaxation, but to choose activities that also address your emotional and mental health.

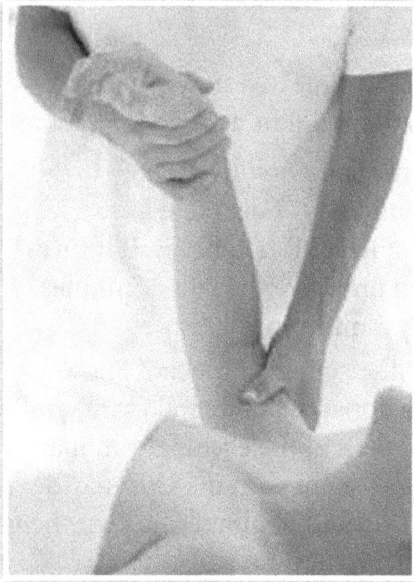

To clarify, the quality of YOU time should be healing to your soul, soothing to your emotions, calming to your mental thoughts, and refreshing to your spirit. That doesn't mean it has to be *all* candles and bubble baths— it can be a vigorous run around the neighborhood if that relaxes you mentally and emotionally.

If you are highly stressed right before YOU time, pulled out a notepad and write down what is really bothering you or heavy on your mind. Then fold the notepad up, put it away—intentionally push that concern from your thoughts, and go enjoy YOU time. Your brain can relax knowing it has documented that concern, so it's fine for you to leave it behind.

One final comment—it's probably a good idea to talk to your partner before starting YOU time, so that they understand what you are doing. Men, in particular, often tend to struggle with understanding the importance of nurturing mental and emotional health, but telling them *why* is better than just surprising them with what they might simply see as "selfish ME" time. Explain that you will also be sharing more time with them and the kids soon as well, because you want to invest that time with your family. If nothing else, feel free to share the first few pages of this chapter to read; it might help your partner understand how a few minutes of quiet sanity for you has happy, healthy benefits for the whole family!

Special Rules for YOU Time

Taking care of yourself does not happen by accident; it's something you must set aside time to do. With this in mind, it is recommended that you communicate that unless someone is actually hurt or the house is burning down, that as an adult, you need 15 minutes of time to yourself with *no interruptions.* If your kids are younger and your spouse can watch the kids, then make that arrangement (and return the favor if you've both been working), or send the kids to their rooms (use a monitor for the youngest ones) if they tend to get into trouble when left together and alone.

Interruptions for silly reasons should result in discipline of whatever nature you deem appropriate; the point is that the kids should understand this time is sacred to you. And because you will also eventually (if you are not now) be spending dedicated time with each child, the kids should mature through the process to understand that this is your time, and they will also get time with you later.

Here are a few suggestions of activities which—when done correctly—nurture the emotions and mental health, as well as the physical body. Don't get stuck into doing one or two things all the time—variety is the spice of life, and much like a variety of foods offers increased nutrients to the body, a variety of experiences offers healthy benefits as well!

INVEST TIME in YOURSELF

- Activity ideas for YOU time:
- Meditating on something happy or positive, or perhaps a scripture verse
- Journaling 3 positive things you were grateful for that day
- Online shopping for something new
- Experiment with a new hairstyle
- Enjoy a body scrub and shower
- Oil treatment for hair or skin
- Write a poem or a song
- Manicure or pedicure
- Read a good book
- Call a friend
- Exercise
- Prayer

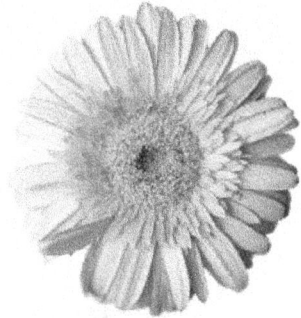

Whatever you choose, do the activity because you want to do it, and not because you feel you have to do it. It must be pleasurable to you, so don't pick something you don't like. As you spend this time on YOU, if your mind wanders, think about the things that happened that day which were happy or positive. These happy thoughts can be accomplishments, or something that someone else did that makes you smile. Release negative thoughts immediately.

Be prepared that, as you start this habit, you may find that this activity feels like *one more burden* to add to your day. It's sad that people sometimes feel this way, but it happens. A little time spent on you should *never* feel like a burden. Let me share with you the truth: if you are having that thought, it's because you are already mentally or emotionally worn out. Stick with this habit and you will eventually find that the nurturing you give yourself during this time will ease the overall stress levels in your life. Eventually you will look forward to YOU time every day, and it won't feel like a burden.

REFERENCE	LOCATION
Skincare recipes	159

○ NURTURING OTHERS

A happy, healthy lifestyle includes embracing relationships with others. Today's world is so busy that valuing and nurturing relationships does not occur by accident. No doubt you have loved ones who you enjoy spending time with, so this section is to help you balance that time with the other things going on in your life.

Time with Your Partner

This time is dedicated to providing loving support to your spouse or partner, and to ensure you communicate on a regular basis. You are each other's support team; view this time as investing in your support. Sharing concerns is normal, but try not to make it a 'vent session'; instead, take turns talking and listening. Be a good listener, and be supportive. This is a no fighting zone!

0

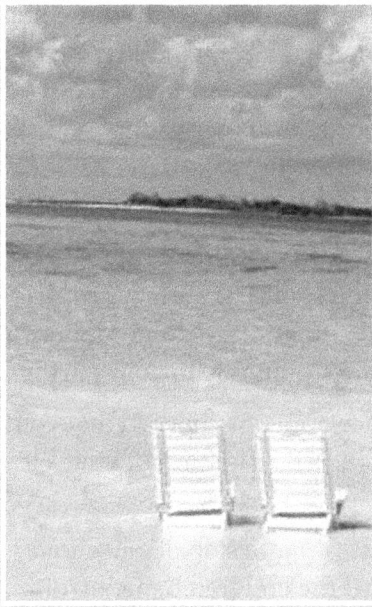

It is particularly true that male partners sometimes complain (fairly or unfairly) that once they had kids, the kids became the higher priority in the life of their female partner, and they feel like yesterday's leftovers. Regardless of the reason for the perception—because in the end, the details don't matter on this—dedicating just this small amount of time to your partner each day will correct this issue or prevent it from ever becoming a problem in your relationship. It cements intimacy and closeness between the two of you. Retreat to your bedroom or the back deck, wherever you can get 15 minutes away from the kids, and spend some quality time together.

As with YOU time, the rule for the kids should be 'no interruptions'! If preferred, this time can be spent after the kids have been tucked into bed, but this should only be done if the two of you are still awake and alert enough to enjoy quality time together, including sex.

- Activity ideas for time with your partner:
- Give each other a foot rub or back massage with peppermint oil or lavender oil
- Genuine conversation (catch up on your day, concerns, etc.)
- Move that conversation to creative spots to 'get away'—on the back porch with a glass of wine, in the car in the driveway, with a prepared snack, etc.
- Enjoy smoothies with maca powder—a healthy and natural aphrodisiac
- Walk around the block or at a nearby park
- Cuddling
- Sex

It is also important to occasionally supplement this time with something more. Leave each other little thank you notes or send a text message saying *I love you*. It's also good to get away a bit longer when you can—go out on date night for dinner or a movie (or both!), or take an occasional holiday away together. If you have kids, hire a babysitter, or make arrangements with another family to watch your kids one weekend, and you return the favor for them another time. Invest in each other.

Previously I mentioned that time with the spouse is a higher priority than the kids. I mean this with all reasonable intentions—do not ignore a genuinely hurting child in favor of spending its 15 minutes with your partner.

Instead, what this means is that you display for your children that your relationship with your spouse is extremely important to both of you. This has several very important, even life-long implications for all:

1. Time invested in each other provides a more stable household foundation for the entire family, and the children benefit from that.

2. Your children will grow up to have relationships where they imitate your family structure. If you are too busy to spend time with your partner, they will subconsciously fall into those same habits when they grow up because it was what they witnessed at home. Therefore, spending time and investing in a happy relationship is critical—the higher you set the bar in your own relationship, you can be assured that your children will set the bar high when choosing their own partner.

A solid home life is something that will reap rewards in the lives of your children many times over.

Time with Your Kids

The time spent with your kids is investing in their well-being, health, and ensuring they feel loved and safe in the home. Just as you give 15 minutes to yourself and to your partner, give that time to your kids as well. It is also recommended that each of the parents (where possible) spend 5 minutes of this daily time with the kids, separately, alone with each kid. If one parent is particularly stressed with work, then it would be okay for them to do this activity once or twice a week, as long as the other partner has the ability to do it daily.

This time spent separately with each parent is to ensure the child that they are important to both of you, and that each of them are uniquely loved. Also, spending time alone is critical, because the child may share things with you (worries, fears) that they may be too embarrassed to share with their siblings around, or with the other parent.

Don't pressure your child to speak. Simply let them know that they have 5 minutes with you each night, just the two of you, where you can talk about whatever they like—happy stuff or sad stuff. Tucking them into bed might be the ideal time to do this.

Aside from this critical few minutes spent with each child, get involved in what your kids love as well as broadening their horizons! If kids spent more time being challenged to learn new things at home, they are less likely to be as curious about other things they shouldn't be (i.e., drugs and alcohol). Wear out their curiosity!

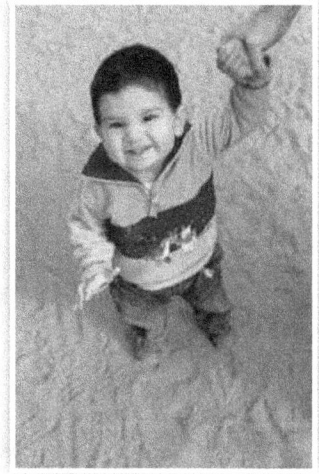

- Activity ideas for time with your kids:
- game night
- hiking or camping
- time at the park
- bedtime stories
- going to a museum
- writing stories together and sharing them
- cooking together (or sharing another life skill)

The worksheet you completed at the opening of this chapter included a short list of life skills for teaching your kids, such as cooking, ironing, mending clothes, etc. Generations ago, it was expected that parents would teach their kids how to complete these 'life skills', but it might be tempting today to think that whatever your kids don't know, they will just research on the internet.

That is true in some ways, but it also misses the point. Teaching your kids these skills is important for their development, their independence, and maturity! It's probably been a while since some of us were kids, so it might be hard to remember what it was like to first learn how to balance a chequebook or refill fluids in a car. It can be confusing; after all, it's not something we are born knowing.

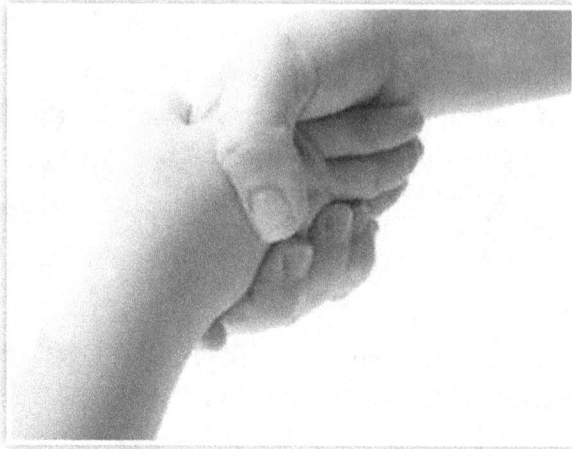

While your kids may complain at first, I strongly believe they will come to appreciate this time together. Choose life skill activities that are age appropriate and then pair them with outings you know they will love more (teaching balancing the chequebook before going to the zoo, for example). As always, use this time to be open with your kids and ask how they are doing without being pushy.

An extra benefit of teaching life skills is that moving forward they can then help you with these activities around the house. You face less of a burden on you or your partner. When you're kids are ready to leave the home, you won't have to guess—you will *know* they are ready for the 'real world'!

Time with Others

Outside of your immediate family, no doubt you have friends and family that you enjoy spending time with. You probably even have some family and friends that you don't enjoy spending time with, but do so anyway. Everybody has personality conflicts with somebody, and that really doesn't change as we get older. While you might have to endure time with some, you likely also have family and friends that you love and wish you could see more of.

For those who are close by, hopefully you get a chance to see your friends or family on a fairly regular basis such as holidays. If you are a good planner, hopefully you get time for a girls night (or guys night) every now and then. If so, consider yourself blessed!

This is a more difficult task for those who have friends or family who live further away. Many get caught into the trap of only seeing each other when a funeral happens (not the happiest of circumstances to catch up with people). Consider planning an informal family reunion so that everyone has a good excuse for getting together for a *happy* reason! If you need to travel, pick a location where a mini vacation could happen at the same time, and you might be able to fill two needs at once.

Even if your family or friends are far from you, hopefully you still pick up the phone or send an email to them. Social media has its faults, but it certainly can help you to stay current with events in the lives of those you love, so you might consider a Facebook account just for that purpose, if you don't have one already.

Aside from friends and family, many people find volunteering to be an activity that is beneficial to their own lives. They enjoy the opportunity to partner with an organization that allows them to meet others, donating their time or other resources to help. Not only does this make you a valuable member of the community but it is a tremendous example to your children. If that is something you have a desire to get involved in, perhaps now might be the time to jump in!

○ LIVING A RICH LIFE

This chapter wouldn't be complete with talking about the value of adding rich experiences to our lives—the kind of experiences we often talk about doing but rarely ever do. The ones that we could do if put effort toward it, but we often let busyness in our lives drown out the desire to try something more.

Wherever you are in your life right now, is there something you've always wanted to do, but have either lacked the resources or the courage to do it? As humans, we have dreams. Those dreams that are positive should be nurtured. Thinking back, even as children, if we had encouraging parents we probably felt no limitations when we thought about the future.

Food For Health
TURNING THE FOOD PYRAMID ON ITS HEAD

Eventually time and experience teaches us that certain jobs or choices are more practical, and for the sake of our security we move toward them—and likely they were the best choice for the time and circumstance.

However, that doesn't mean that we shouldn't enjoy a life where we experience some of those positive desires of our heart! For example have you ever wanted to:

- Learn another language
- Explore a foreign country
- Become a connoisseur of wine or coffee
- Take a course to further your education—or learn something new
- Start a new project around the house (something you've never done before)
- Take a hot air balloon ride
- Go bungee jumping
- Parachute from an aeroplane

These are fantastic dreams! They stir up interest in your life, giving you a passion and a focus, plus they also provide experiences that provoke conversation between you and your partner or you and your friends. *That is what living a healthy lifestyle looks like.*

No one is suggesting you pick a hobby and pursue it like Captain Ahab after Moby Dick—just enjoy it in balance with the rest of your life. Still others who believe they want to live a fun dramatic life think that means heading to a club to get drunk every weekend. That is the *opposite* of living a rich and dramatic life! Drinking can be very enjoyable, but what's fun about having a weekend you won't even remember later? Instead, live a life that has you reaching for the stars in a healthy way.

Perhaps you are thinking that this type of thought process is ridiculous—that only kids have dreams and that you had to

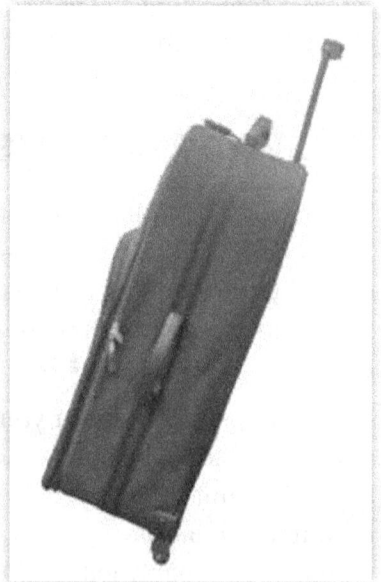

stop your dreaming years ago. Stop and tell yourself right now: *if you want something bad enough, you can make it happen*, and that is a good thing. The world needs more dreamers and action takers! The human spirit thrives on dreams.

It might be difficult. It might take years of preparation depending on how big the dream is. But if you make the decisions now that will put you on the path to what you want, *you can do it*. You only get one shot at life, so live a life that will make you smile!

○ **TAKE ACTION**

Day 5 should be inspirational to you! You *can* live a life that nurtures you and all the relationships in your life with only a little effort—it just requires the right balance of priorities. You can also live a life that dreams big! So don't live the life others tell you; live the life *you* were meant to live.

Step 1. Make a list of all the important people in your life—relationships that you want to invest in.

Step 2. Start by investing in YOU time today!

Step 3. Add the other relationships in order of priority.

Step 4. Write down a list of your dreams and make plans to start on one of them within the next month.

Only two days left! Now it's time for Day 6.

DAY 6:
Family Budget

6

"A budget is telling your money where to go instead of wondering where it went."

~ **Ramsey** ~

ONEY IS USUALLY NOT a pleasant subject. Many times you don't have enough of it, and everybody always wants more of it no matter how much they currently have now.

To add to the complications, most families have one adult that loves to save (or spend more conservatively) while another adult tends to view money as a commodity that should be spent and enjoyed. This clash of world views or perspectives can cause friction in the family unit.

But who's right?

○ CHALLENGES OF LIVING ON A BUDGET

The truth is that with money there is no right or wrong in the details. It isn't that you can't buy this dress or whether he should buy that expensive pair of shoes or not. Both adults are aware that money is valuable to the safety of the family unit. Both would agree that living without a roof over their heads would be difficult and hazardous to the safety of everyone. The big problem is that the two adults do not have one goal about family needs and how to plan for them financially.

- When faced with buying decisions, the only two questions really should be:
- Do we physically have money in the bank to spend?

If we have the money, where should we be spending it?

And to answer the second question, you need to have a budget.

Identify Unhealthy Financial Habits

It's time to examine your current spending habits! Take a few minutes to examine the status of the family's finances.

REFERENCE	LOCATION
Identify Your Unhealthy Financial Habits	161

After you have completed the worksheet, total up your responses. How did you do?

Reject Unhealthy Financial Habits

Did you score better or worse than you thought? Some will score well on most of the responses; however, in the end if you are not saving or putting away money for retirement, you could still be in trouble *tomorrow* if you fail to put your affairs into order today.

That's living life on a gamble.

Don't wait for disaster to strike. Take advantage of the time you have now to move yourself into a better position financially. Your stress levels will dramatically reduce when money problems are out of the picture. You will sleep better at night knowing your bills are paid for and your children are being taken care of. Even if you honestly feel you don't make enough money to make ends meet, there are things you can do to improve your situation.

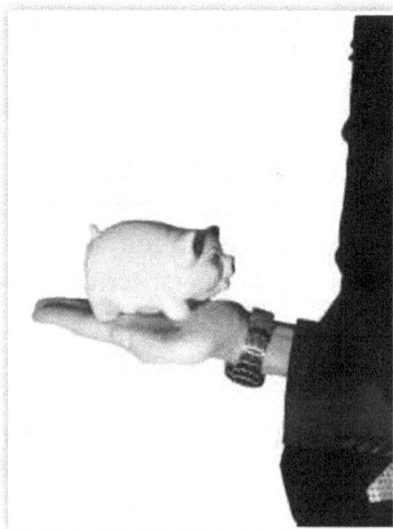

But you have to make a decision that the only acceptable way is to live life in the 'black' and not the 'red'.

Choose Healthy Financial Habits

The only way to make better financial decisions is to know exactly where you stand. You've answered the worksheet so you have a better idea of your general financial habits, but we need to dig deeper.

Everyone knows the only way to come out on top financially is to make more money than you spend. It's simple math. You can do this a few different ways:

- Option 1. You make so much money that you require little awareness of your budget to live financially free.
- Option 2. You make enough money to pay the bills, or even a little extra, but you have to watch your budget to ensure you don't overspend.
- Option 3. You are required to pinch and scrape on costs in order to keep your head above water.

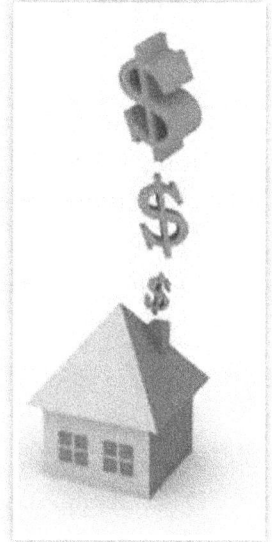

Most of us will not find ourselves in the first option. Most of use will fit into options 2 or 3, and we will benefit from taking a good hard look at our financial numbers and living a bit more simply. Even if you don't make enough money to pay the bills, chances are your situation can be improved with a few decisions tied to a few basic concepts.

With that in mind, all it takes to reverse your situation is a decision to live more financially wise.

Commitment 6: **Choose to live by a budget until you are living financially free.**

The concept of living financially free will be more defined in the next section, but everyone has the ability to make this choice. Are you ready to do what it takes to live financially free?

Food For Health

○ THE ROAD TO FINANCIAL FREEDOM

Moving from financial prison to financial freedom is possible. It requires a commitment to *want* to be successful, which goes beyond just wanting to make money. Success is more than just money—it involves living by a set of rules where you choose to do the right thing. Living smart to make smart money. Don't skip out on paying the toll fee. Don't try to avoid the speeding ticket. Making bad choices often comes with financial penalties—get organized, do the right thing, and the extra costs will reduce.

It also means that to get to the point of being successful, you must exercise self-discipline to save on costs and live on a budget. This is not an easy thing, because it isn't a one-time decision; you must choose to live on a restricted budget with every choice you make for an extended amount of time. It will not happen overnight.

Being financially free means:

- you can pay your bills
- you know how to pay off unavoidable debts (i.e., house mortgages)
- you have a minimum of 3 months of savings in your account
- you have a sizable nest age saved for retirement

The first step is understanding where you are financially.

Crunch the Numbers

First things first—you must be aware of your income, bills, and other expenses, or you will not be able to dig yourself out of any financial hole you might be in. To get a good grasp of where you are, pull out your most recent bills, bank statements, receipts, and payment stubs, print the form below and complete it. You'll have to crunch some numbers. It's time to evaluate your cash flow!

REFERENCE	LOCATION
Your Family Budget	162

After you have completed the form, you aren't done yet! Once you have the numbers in place, now is the important step—evaluating where you can make changes.

Evaluate Your Results

What was your final number? Did you come out on top, or are you in the red financially?

It's time to evaluate. You must reduce your debt, and by doing so, the money you make will go further!

- Ideas for short term options to reduce expenses include:
- lowering electricity costs by keeping the windows open more often
- choose to use a clothesline rather than a dryer
- sell an unnecessary vehicle, stocks, or other assets.
- host a yard sale

Some efforts might not bring in much, but they should be considered because every bit of money gets you closer to your goal.

Not only can you often cut back on short term expenses, but for long term cost reduction, consider the chapter on sustainability. Can you grow more of your own food? Produce and eat more fermented foods or sprout your own vegies? While the savings may not be felt immediately, they cost little to implement and are healthy choices for your wallet.

You can also try ideas to increase your income including:

- investment in an income property
- setting up an online business
- joining an MLM company
- investing in shares with a friend
- making crafts with your kids and placing the items for sale on Etsy or Ebay
- completing online surveys
- offering to do the laundry and ironing for a busy family
- cleaning homes or mowing lawns in the neighborhood
- asking for a raise at your current job

Finally, consider a different viewpoint when making purchases. It's normal to expect to take on debt for a house, and occasionally a vehicle. However, even with vehicle and home purchases, large down payments should be saved up before purchase to reduce the amount of interest paid;

this offers you savings felt over the life of the loan. Once you do take on a loan, plan to pay more than the monthly payment amount in order to end the loan faster.

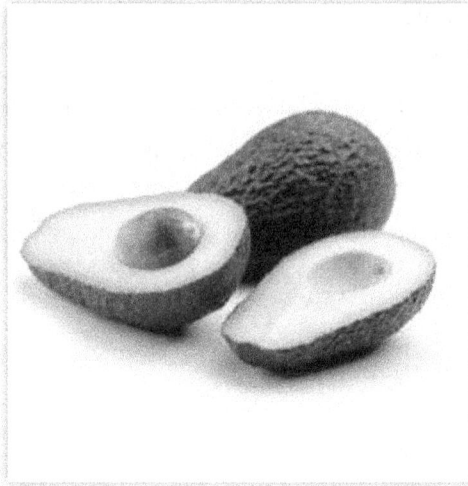

Payments for clothes, appliances, and other household goods should not be paid on credit unless you plan to pay them off immediately, and finally, always shop smart—be patient and use sales and coupons to reduce your costs. Get to know your local grocery stores; compare prices on the foods and pantry items you are buying and see where it is the smartest to shop. Use the handout below to help you compare prices spent at your local stores like Coles and Woolworths.

REFERENCE	LOCATION
Grocery Store Comparison Chart	xx

A few additional rules to consider when making purchases:

- Only spend money you have—do not spend money on credit that you cannot pay off immediately
- When you do spend money on credit, pay it off before the next pay cycle or when interest is added
- Call your credit card company to ask if you can have payments moved or even temporarily halted (not all will do this, but it is worth your time to call and find out)

- Always be up front and communicate with your creditors—they will be more likely to work with you

Finalize Your Budget

Once you have spoken with your creditors, determined where adjustments can be made to spending, and have sold any assets you can to reduce debt, you now have a monthly budget. Complete your budget spreadsheet again with your new numbers, and monitor your progress each and every month.

Once you have your completed spreadsheet, it's important to share the results with the rest of the family, including the kids. Why? Well, you're all in the same boat together. Kids know when the truth is being withheld from them, and they also may grow bitter or frustrated if you tell them 'no' on purchases without giving them a *why*. If you are in dire financial straits, you don't have to share all the details, but it is important the kids have at least a basic understanding if money is tight or worse.

Once your budget is finalized, you are on your way to financial freedom, because the first step is knowledge, and the second step is commitment. Take back control! Make the changes necessary, and with time, you will soon avoid the pinch of no money.

However, be sure that your plans to financial freedom include a sizeable savings account for emergencies, as well as saving for retirement. Until those issues are resolved, you are still living at risk of falling back into a money trap.

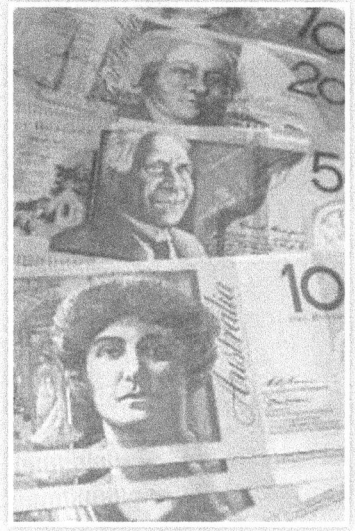

○ TAKE ACTION

Day 6 can be tough! No one wants to think about money or whether we are living beyond our means. However, choosing to living a life committed to financial freedom puts you in better control of your family's future.

Food For Health

Step 1. Print out the "Your Family Budget" sheet and complete with your *final* monthly totals.

Step 2. Label the fifth divider "Family Budget" and insert your newly printed sheets there.

Step 3. Evaluate your budget every month, and as you reduce debt, share the progress with the family. The progress will be motivating to everyone!

Your final day is in front of you: Day 7!

DAY 7:
Routines

7

"Routine is a ground to stand on, a wall to retreat to; we cannot draw on our boots without bracing ourselves against it."

~ David Thoreau ~

O<small>N</small> D<small>AY</small> 1, I mentioned there was a big secret that was key to everything in this book.

"There is one big secret to all of this. One thing that is a huge game changer as you move forward. It draws the line in the sand between success and failure."

Have you been able to guess what that secret is?

It's *action*.

The line between success and failure is taking action. You must be willing to move to get the changes done. For example, I can read about gardening all day, even for years, but if I never plant a seed all I've done is take in knowledge. I am not a gardener. I could be one if I chose, because I possess the knowledge, but I am not one until I take the action.

Take action can be difficult at times, but we can make the fight a little bit easier by working smarter rather than harder. We can do that by having a routine in place for all the things we love—or need—to do.

○ LOVING THE ROUTINE

*Routine...*even the very name sounds so dull. Who would want to live a *routine life*? A routine existence? Why do the same thing day in and day out?

There are certainly aspects of routine that are hum-drum and dull. A boring life should make you want to run screaming! And it is also certainly true that a life *full* of routine is not really a life at all. As mentioned in Day 5, living a life that is rich in love, relationships, and experience is far more satisfying to the soul and mind than a life of dullness.

However, there are routines which are very beneficial. Certain routines, when done appropriately and correctly, allow us to achieve balance in our lives while having the time to *live* our lives. These are the routines we have discussed throughout the course of this book and which help us to build good habits.

When left to chance—or our frazzled minds—we will not always remember to water the garden when we should. We may overlook the kid's theatre performance, or when to pay the water bill. Our friend may invite us to dinner but we forget to buy the ingredients to make a delicious dish to bring, so we rush to the store to buy something last minute—not near as yummy or healthy—and we arrive harried and tired.

No matter what society might say, completely winging life isn't fun.

There's no need to go to extremes. Certainly no one needs to plan out every minute of their day or every second of a party, for example—you just need to be sure you remember the important things.

Now, each chapter (day) of this book had its own recommendations for little routines, but there is only one way to coordinate everything and ensure you make it to where you need to be, and on time. Your final two tools are below.

REFERENCE	LOCATION
Calendar, Daily "To Do" List	170

With these two tools, you can get organized! These are the final pieces. Keep it simple and you are more likely to remember to use them.

Calendar

This particular handout is not provided in the book because including a specific calendar year would require regular updates to the book; plus, this is a resource easily found online.

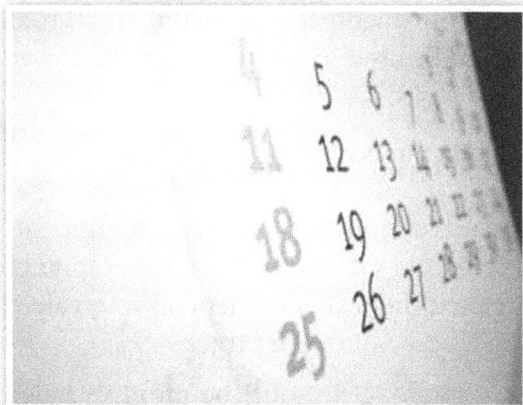

Search for blank calendars that allow you to print for the current calendar year, in the format you desire, and include holiday dates if you wish. Then print and hole punch for your binder.

Once printed, document the following on them:

- Birthdays, anniversaries, and other special family events
- School and after-school events
- Menu planning and grocery shopping (include time to ferment vegies, sprout, etc.)
- Time for working in the garden or yard
- Time for housecleaning
- Time for YOU, family, friends, and activities
- Time for balancing the budget and paying the bills

Once a week, spending a few minutes reviewing the upcoming week events to see if anything needs to be added or adjusted.

Daily "To Do" List

Print out the form and insert it in a sheet protector; then place it in the binder at the very front. Use a wet erase texta to write on *top* of the protector but 'inside' the blanks to fill out the form each day, and wipe with a damp paper towel or cloth to erase—this allows you to reuse the same sheet each day.

While your calendar allows you to get to do high level planning for the future, your "Daily 'To Do' List" helps you decide what to do each new day, allowing you to break off your big goals into small chunks of activity.

Both documents fill an important role in keeping you coordinated and should be used in conjunction with one another.

O TAKE ACTION

You're working on your final commitment—and it's a critical one! Without this step, all of your mini-routines might feel a little chaotic as you try to organize them all. Put them on your calendar and "Daily 'To Do' List" and you'll keep yourself on track!

Step 1. Print out the monthly calendars and complete with your routines and special events, as described above.

Step 2. Label the FIRST divider "Family Calendar" and insert the calendars behind this tab.

Step 3. Print out the "Daily 'To Do' List", insert in a sheet protector, and write on top of the sheet protector with a wet erase texta to complete it each evening for the next day.

Step 4. Place this sheet *before* the first divider. It should be the first thing you see when you open the binder.

FINAL THOUGHTS

8

Q UITE OFTEN, CHANGE COMES about in our lives because of tragedy. However, in this case you have a valuable opportunity to start over without the prompting of a terrible cause. Grab it. While you will not be able to do everything at once, you can make dramatic changes that set your life on a very positive course.

No one is judging you on what you do. In the end, you can only change if you want to change. Make these changes because you see the value in them and you realize that positive change brings positive results.

This takes on even more meaning if you have children, who will grow up in your footsteps and will live a life that in many ways emulates yours. If you had the power to choose for them, would you give them the life you have now...or would you give them more?

Best wishes and good health to you and your family!

Samantha Baird

APPENDIX A

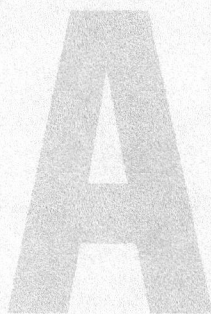

A

Identify Your Food Habits

1. Describe your childhood mealtimes. What were common foods on the table? Did you eat out a lot?

2. Who taught you about nutrition and eating habits as you grew up?

3. Do you identify with the eating habits of any of your family members?

4. Is there a history of any chronic health diseases or other health issues in your family? List them here and be detailed. Include surgeries and medications for managing symptoms. If possible, talk to family members to be sure you have a very clear picture of the health issues your family has struggled with.

5. What are your current health complaints?

6. Create a list of your recent meals. If you can remember the meals you have eaten the last few days, feel free to include them; otherwise, start today and write them down before our next consultation.

Date	Meal	Food

7. Do you see any correlation between bad food choices in the past, and your health problems today? Talk to me about these results.

RAW FOODS: Eating Plan Breakdown

Raw Food Eating Choices

Raw foods focuses on eating healthy organic whole foods in their natural raw state. If you choose a raw foods diet (also called being a raw foodie) you can enjoy the following foods:

- Raw vegies
- Raw fruits
- Beans
- Cacao
- Sprouts from seed, nut, grain, or bean sources
- Roots such as beetroot and ginger
- Avocado, nuts, and seeds (eat some at every meal)
- Oils
- Cooked legumes and potatoes (only once a week)

> *Supplement water with a slice of lemon in the morning, and a teaspoon of apple cider vinegar before dinner.*

Cooking Rules

- The majority of your food should be eaten in its raw state
- Occasionally steaming food is fine
- Never cook above 46 degrees to protect the nutrients

Food Prep Tools

- Reliable cooking thermometer to monitor temperature
- Dehydrator
- Food processor
- Blender
- Clean with apple cider vinegar

DIRTY PRODUCE Buy Organic

Popular fruits and vegies that are considered to be the most contaminated with pesticides:

- Apples
- Celery
- Cherry tomatoes
- Cucumber
- Grapes
- Hot peppers
- Nectarines (imported)
- Peaches
- Potatoes
- Spinach
- Strawberries
- Sweet capsicum
- Kale / collard greens
- Summer squash

> *When choosing your produce, eat a lot of green, but always choose a mix of the remaining vegie color categories: yellow & orange, blue & purple, red, and white.*

CLEAN PRODUCE Organic or Non-Organic

Popular fruits and vegies that are considered to be the least contaminated with pesticides:

- Asparagus
- Avocados
- Cabbage
- Rock melon
- Sweet corn
- Aubergines (eggplant)
- Grapefruit
- Kiwi
- Mangos
- Mushrooms
- Papayas
- Pineapples
- Sweet peas (frozen)
- Sweet potatoes

RAW VEGIE PROTEIN: Cheat Sheet

P ROTEIN IS AN IMPORTANT macronutrient for living a healthy lifestyle, and the good news is that you can boost your protein numbers through vegies alone. Take this list with you when you go grocery shopping to help plan your meals and ensure you get the protein you need!

VEGIE	SERVING SIZE	PROTEIN	CALO-RIES
Sprouts (average)	1 cup / 207g	40g	700
Lentils	.5 cup	24.8g	336
Beans (average)	Varies	12g	148
Cauliflower	1 head / 588g	11g	146
Green Peas	1 cup	8g	118
Spirulina	100g	5.9g	26
Broccoli	148g	4.2g	50
Artichokes	1 artichoke / 128g	4.2g	60
Asparagus	1 spear / 16g	3g	3
Brussels Sprouts	1 cup / 88g	3g	38
Kale	1 cup / 67g	2.9g	33
Sweet Corn, White	1 ear / 90g	2.9g	77
Bok Choy	1 cup / 170g	2.6g	20
Zucchini	1 medium / 196g	2.4g	33
Watercress	100g	2.3g	11

VEGIE	SERVING SIZE	PROTEIN	CALO-RIES
Acorn Squash	1 cup / 245g	1.6g	82
Capsicum	.5 cup / 75g	1.5g	30
Onion	1 medium / 110g	1.2g	44
Cucumber (peeled)	1 medium / 201 g	1.2g	25

Food for health. Food for life! *Food4health.com.au*

Food For Health
TURNING THE FOOD PYRAMID ON ITS HEAD

BLENDER REVIEW

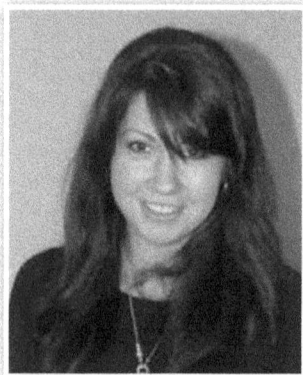

HELLO, I'M SAMANTHA BAIRD, owner *of Food for Health. People frequently ask me for my recommendations on which blender I prefer, so I decided to document my own experience so I could share it with others.*

Hopefully you are considering my recommendation to become a raw foodie! If so, you need a good blender that can support your new lifestyle. Being a food coach, I use my blender for work and home use. It would be an understatement that my blenders get a good work out several times day! This year I have seen myself through a few of these costly items, so I thought it might help to share my results.

One of my first blenders was a basic Breville. It did the job. I found that if I put in something like banana and rice milk, or honey, it was fine; as soon as I added greens or dates, it got lumpy. If you're a smoothie lover like me, lumps are a no-no. What killed my blender was adding ice—one blitz, and it died.

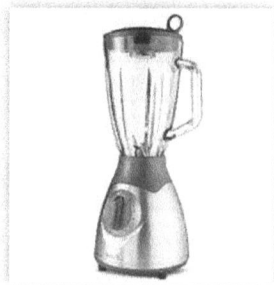

Next I tried a Philips 1000W Compact 3-in-1 Setup 3.4L Bowl Food Processor. Great value for the money, the food processor component of this machine is good. However, the

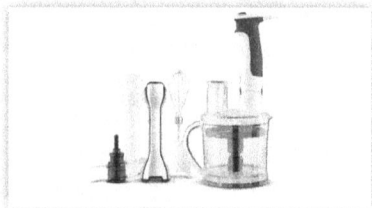

blender can't handle ice , and once again, struggles to blend to a smooth consistency.

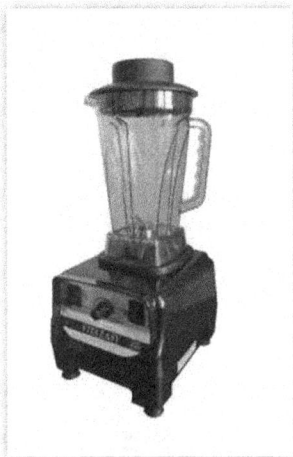

Next was the Breville All-in-One. I love this little device. It's quick and easy, and I still sometime use it for mashed potatoes or will quickly use the stick for my pumpkin soup. However, it isn't very powerful, so you wouldn't use this for a green smoothie.

The Vita Easy was my next large purchase. It's quite expensive (RRP $799.00). This machine is similar to the Vita Mix; you can put in whole foods and blend away! It's a powerful machine. The only downfall is that it doesn't have a switch-off feature, so it can overheat.

My new favourite is the **Optimum 9400** by Froothie. I love this blender! It's reasonably priced under $500—by an Australian company, which is an added bonus. The best part is that when I am making a green smoothie, I can be confident it will come out silky smooth! I put in carrot, beets, zucchini, and greens with ice and it blends easily, no worries. I have also made hot soups, bliss and protein balls, nut butters and milks; this machine does it all! It has a safety cut-off

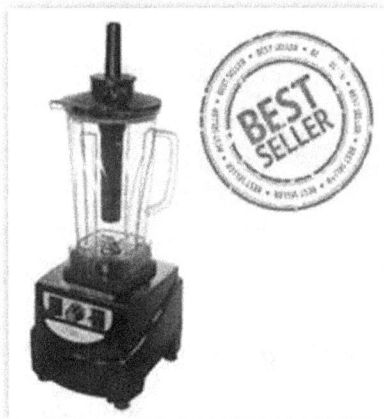

switch, and you can buy an extended warranty, so it is truly a great buy!

No more blowing up blenders for me!

Please contact me if you have any questions!

Samantha Baird

Smoothie Cleanse FAQ

Why should I do a smoothie cleanse?

Consider the benefits...

- Get a boost on your weight loss goals
- Purge stored toxins that can make you feel sluggish or even ill when you exercise
- Enjoy higher energy levels and more vitality for life
- Feel more mentally alert for tackling any of life's problems

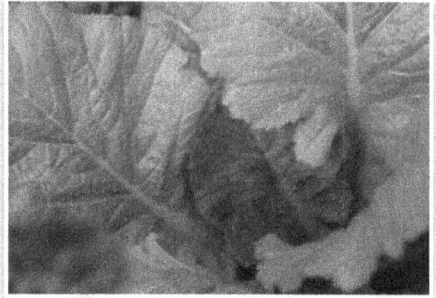

How long should I cleanse?

Most cleanses are recommended on a 5 – 7 or 21 day course. Listen to your body; you will know when your body is ready.

What do I need to complete a smoothie cleanse?

You will need:

- quality vegies
- a good blender (refer to my blender review if you need to purchase one)
- a helpful probiotic (Yor brand recommended; has over 40 billion live microorganisms)
- Yor Super Greens (Maintains an alkaline balance; see my site *www.food4health.com.au* for questions or for convenient purchase)

You might also consider an enema as well, as a gentle way to help assist your body to cleanse.

What should I do once I have completed a cleanse?

Once you have finished your cleanse I recommend you continue for a minimum of 30days on a low stress diet regimen.

What is the best way to build a smoothie with everything I need?

Remember to prepare a good balance of healthy fats, carbohydrates, and proteins in each smoothie you consume! Refer to the Raw Vegie Protein Cheat Sheet for help and then go through the steps below.

1. **Start by choosing a fat source:** nut milk, nuts, seeds, oil such as Udo's, coconut or flax, avocado.
2. **Choose a protein from the chart below.** Also, add a good quality pea protein powder and avoid isolated whey protein; you should remain dairy free while cleansing.
3. **Add a good carb:** banana, dates, pumpkin, sweet potato.
4. **Add your fruit and vegies.** Go nuts and be creative! I love zucchini and banana to add creaminess.
5. **Add fluid:** water, coconut water, coconut milk, nut milk, chilled herbal tea, or ice.
6. **Optional extras:** maca powder, cacao, goji berries, honey, super greens powder, spirullina, chia seeds.
7. Blend and enjoy!

For more information on smoothies, please go to *www.supersmoothiecleanse.com.au*!

This book contains general information about medical conditions and treatments. The information is not advice, and should not be treated as such. The medical information in this book is provided "as is" without any representations or warranties, express or implied. Food for Health makes no representations or warranties in relation to the medical information in this book. Without prejudice to the generality of the foregoing paragraph, Food for Health does not warrant that the medical information in this book will be constantly available, or available at all; or that the medical information in this book is complete, true, accurate, up-to-date, or non-misleading. You must not rely on the information in this book as an alternative to medical advice from your doctor or other professional healthcare provider. If you have any specific questions about any medical matter you should consult your doctor or other professional

A

How to Make a Salad a Complete Meal

healthcare provider. If you think you may be suffering from any medical condition you should seek immediate medical attention. You should never delay seeking medical advice, disregard medical advice, or discontinue medical treatment because of information in this book.

Step 1. Chop up your choice of vegies and/or fruit.

This helps with adequate carbohydrates and energy.

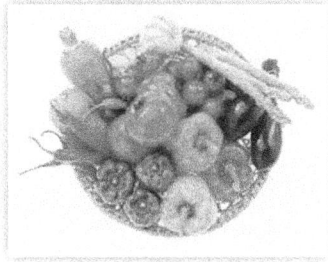

Step 2. Add greens where possible.

Greens have lots of chlorophyll and alkalizing properties.

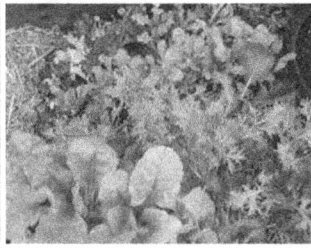

Step 3. Add your protein.

Add some sprouts or corn for a protein boost.. Refer to the "Raw Vegie Protein Cheat Sheet" for helpful suggestions.

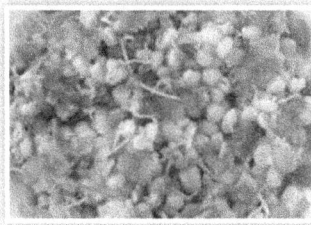

Step 4. Add your fat.

Fat ensures you feel satisfied and helps curb cravings. Olives, flax seed oils, nuts, seeds, and avocado are all good options. Refer to the "Dietary Fats" handout for more information.

Food For Health

RAW FOODS
EATING PLAN:
Breakdown

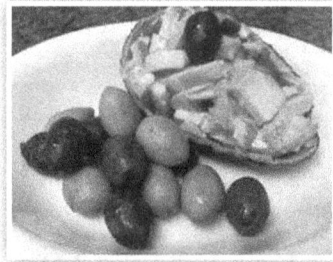

Preparing salads with regards to the components listed above will ensure your salads are healthy and filling enough for a full meal!

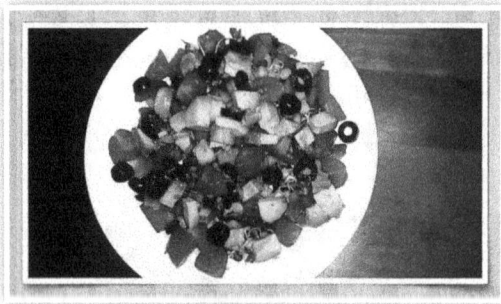

Raw Plus Paleo Eating Choices

Raw foods focuses on eating healthy organic whole foods in their natural raw state. Paleo diet also includes healthy, lean, grass-fed, free-range meats. If you choose the RPP diet you can enjoy the following foods:

- Raw vegies and raw fruits
- Beans
- Cacao
- Sprouts from seed, nut, grain, or bean sources
- Roots such as beetroot and ginger
- Nuts
- Oils
- Cooked legumes and potatoes (two - three times per week)
- Seafood
- Eggs
- Grass-fed, free range meats and wild game

RPP Excludes

- dairy
- cereal grains
- refined sugars
- salt
- processed foods
- refined vegetable oils
- minimal bacon unless nitrate free

> *Supplement water with a slice of lemon in the morning, and a teaspoon of apple cider vinegar before dinner.*

Weekly Schedule

On the RPP plan you eat according the following schedule:

- Raw foods 1 – 2 days each week

- Paleo 5 – 6 days each week
- All meals should include a raw food component
- Organic, free-range chicken eggs, as well as fish, can be eaten as a healthy option at any meal

> *Follow the "Raw Food Eating Plan Breakdown" sheet for help on raw food days. Always choose a mix of the vegie color categories: green, yellow & orange, blue & purple, red, and white.*

Animal Protein Comparison for 100g Servings (3.5 oz)

- Fillet steak, grilled—29g
- Minced, cooked beef—25g
- Sirloin, roasted—32g
- Lamb cutlets, grilled—28g
- Lamb leg, roasted—31g
- Lamb chops, grilled—29g
- Pork fillet, grilled—33g
- Pork leg, roasted—35g
- Pork chop, grilled—32g
- Veal, pan-fried—33g
- Venison, roasted—36g
- Chicken breast, roasted—25g
- Snapper fillet—26g
- Mahi-mahi fillet—18g
- Flathead fillet—26g
- Barramundi fillet—25g
- Sole fillet—21g
- Flounder fillet—21g
- Tuna—22g
- Shrimp—20g
- Egg—13g

9 Day 'Get Started' Meal Plan

A

MEAL	Breakfast	Snack	Lunch	Snack	Dinner
Day 1	Spanish Omelet	Apple	Tuna Wraps	Curried Seeds	Quinoa Curry
Day 2	Spanish Omelet	Apple	Tuna Wraps	Curried Seeds	Quinoa Curry
Day 3	Smoothie	Curried Seeds	Sushi	Mandarin	Chow Mein
Day 4	Smoothie	Curried Seeds	Sushi	Mandarin	Chow Mein
Day 5	Easy Brekky Muffins	Apple	Chicken Salad	Curried Seeds	Tuna Bake
Day 6	Easy Brekky Muffins	Apple	Chicken Salad	Curried Seeds	Tuna Bake
Day 7	Smoothie	Curried Seeds	Ham Wraps	6× Brazil Nuts	Roast Lamb & Veg
Day 8	Smoothie	Curried Seeds	Ham Wraps	6× Brazil Nuts	Roast Lamb & Veg
Day 9	Fruit Salad with Seeds	1 Boiled Egg	Smoothie	6× Brazil Nuts	Roast Veg Soup

Recipes and shopping list are available in Appendix B.

A Elimination Diet for Gluten

To find out if you are gluten intolerant or sensitive, one option is to eliminate all wheat, barley, and rye products from your diet for 1 month. Gluten can be found in any processed food, including raw meat (if stored in broth or caramel colouring), ice cream, and seasoning. Review the "Gluten Free Ingredients List" cheat sheet for help in identifying ingredients on labels which may contain gluten.

Avoid the following:

- Bread of all kinds
- Rice, plain rice crackers
- Cookies, muffins, biscuits
- Cake, pastries
- White sauce
- Processed foods containing wheat (unless labeled gluten-free)
- Ice cream
- Rye, barley, oats
- Corn products of all kinds
- Beer
- Vodka

Eat the following:

- Gluten-free bread (small amounts)
- Gluten-free cookies or biscuits (small amounts)
- Gluten-free pasta (small amounts)

- Oats (if pre-soaked the night before and if rolled or groats, not instant)
- Potatoes, sweet potato, pumpkin
- Fruits
- Vegies
- Raw meats (if they are not stored in broth or caramel colouring)
- Eggs

> *Call the product manufacturer anytime you are uncertain if a product contains gluten (wheat, barley, or rye).*

Elimination Diet

- It is critical you eat completely and strictly wheat/barley/rye free for 1 month.
- You may feel headaches, joint pain, or abdominal pain during withdrawal.
- Write down symptoms experienced during the month, including headaches, tummy pain, joint pain, diarrhoea, constipation, mood swings, irritability, depression, fatigue, mouth ulcers, etc.
- After completing 1 month eating wheat/barley/rye free, complete the 3 Day Challenge (below).

3 Day Challenge

- Eat 6 slices of bread per day (or equivalent) for 3 consecutive days.
- Write down all symptoms for 10 days. Symptoms may be immediate or delayed for a few days.

Day	Symptom
_____	_____
_____	_____
_____	_____
_____	_____

Food For Health
TURNING THE FOOD PYRAMID ON ITS HEAD

GLUTEN FREE: Ingredients List

A gluten-free diet is the only treatment for coeliac disease. Taking gluten out of the diet allows your gut to heal and your symptoms to improve.

Gluten is a protein found in:

- Wheat (including spelt)
- Rye
- Barley
- Oats
- Pasta
- Processed foods
- White sauce made from flour
- Noodles
- Lollies, ice-cream candy
- Some soups and ice cream

Foods that are safe to eat:

- Naturally gluten free foods. For example: Fresh fruit and vegetables, fresh meats, eggs, nuts and legumes, milk, fats and oils, and gluten free grains, e.g., rice and corn.
- Products labelled 'gluten free'. You can be confident that products displaying the 'gluten free' label are safe.
- Products that use the 'Crossed grain logo'. Products displaying the crossed grain logo are endorsed by Coeliac Australia and are safe.

- Products that are gluten free by ingredient. If any ingredient in a product is derived from wheat, rye, barley or oats, then this must be declared.

Gluten Ingredients (always avoid)

- Barley Malt
- Beer (most contain barley or wheat)
- Bleached flour/Enriched Bleached Flour/Enriched Bleached Wheat Flour
- Bran
- Bread Flour
- Brewer's Yeast
- Rye
- Seitan
- Semolina

Hidden Gluten Ingredients

Call the manufacturer when these ingredients are on a label to clarify if it contains gluten.

- Artificial Colour
- Baking Powder
- Caramel Color
- Caramel Flavouring
- Clarifying Agents
- Coloring
- Dextrins
- Dextrimaltose
- Dry Roasted Nuts
- Emulsifiers
- Enzymes
- Fat Replacer
- Flavoring
- Food Starch
- Food Starch Modified
- Glucose Syrup
- Gravy Cubes
- Ground Spices
- Hydrolyzed Plant Protein (HPP)
- Hydrolyzed Protein
- Hydrolyzed Vegetable Protein (HVP)
- Hydrogenated Starch Hydrolysate
- Hydroxypropylated Starch
- Maltose
- Miso
- Mixed Tocopherols
- Modified Food Starch
- Modified Starch
- Natural Flavouring
- Natural Flavours
- Natural Juices
- Non-dairy Creamer
- Pregelatinized Starch
- Protein Hydrolysates
- Seafood Analogs
- Seasonings
- Sirimi
- Smoke Flavouring
- Soba Noodles

- Soy Sauce
- Soy Sauce Solids
- Sphingolipids
- Stabilizers
- Starch

- Stock Cubes
- Suet
- Tocopherols
- Vegetable Broth
- Vegetable Gum

GLUTEN FREE:
Shopping List

A

SWEETENERS

- Agave syrup
- Raw honey
- Organic maple syrup
- Dark chocolate
- Vanilla extract (check label)

GRAIN

- Rice

SPICES

- Black pepper
- Caraway seeds
- Celtic sea salt
- Cinnamon
- Curry
- Paprika

OILS

- Flaxseed oil
- Grapeseed oil
- Olive oil
- Organic coconut oil
- Sesame oil
- UDO's oil
- Safflower oil
- Cacoa butter

HOW TO USE THIS SHOPPING LIST

Shop smarter and avoid making extra trips!

Print a few of these sheets for your binder.

Circle items when you run out during the week, and go through the list once more before leaving for the grocery.

Scratch items off the list as you buy them.

SEEDS

- Chia
- Linseeds
- Poppy seeds
- Pumpkin/pepitas

- Sesame seeds
- Quinoa seeds
- Tahina
- Wholegrain mustard
- Massel stock - beef, chicken, vegie
- Nama Shoyu/Tamari

VINEGARS

- Apple cider vinegar
- Balsamic vinegar
- Rice wine vinegar

POWDERS

- Acai
- Cacao powder
- Green Qi/Super Greens
- Maca
- Pea protein
- Raw carob powder
- Sea Power/Kelp
- Spirulina
- Almond meal
- Arrowroot
- Baking powder
- Coconut - desiccated, shredded

FLOURS/THICKENERS

- Corn meal/polenta
- Bean flours
- Tapioca flour/starch
- Quinoa flour
- Coconut flour

- Potato flour/starch
- Xanthan gum
- Guar gum
- Pectin

ANIMAL PROTEIN

- Bacon (only nitrate free)
- Beef
- Chicken
- Emu
- Fish
- Kangaroo
- Lamb
- Marrow bones (stock)
- Mince
- Pork
- Sausages (gluten free)
- Shrimp/seafood

BEANS/LEGUMES

- Adzuki beans
- Navy beans
- Baked beans
- Chickpeas (garbanzo)
- Mungbeans (sprouting)
- Lentils
- Red kidney beans

DAIRY

- Eggs
- Yogurt

NUT MILKS

- Almond

- Coconut
- Rice

NUTS

- Almond
- Brazil
- Cashew
- Hazelnut
- Pinenuts
- Pistachio
- Walnut

> The items on this list are traditionally gluten free; however, it is your responsibility to always verify the item does not contain gluten by reading labels and consulting with product manufacturers for confirmation.

FRUIT

- Apples (red , green)
- Bananas
- Coconut
- Grapes
- Honey dew melon
- Kiwi
- Mandarin
- Mango
- Oranges
- Papaya

- Passion fruit
- Pears
- Pineapple
- Rockmelon
- Strawberries
- Watermelon
- Lemon
- Lime

VEGIES

- Asparagus
- Avocados
- Beetroot
- Broccoli
- Brussels sprouts
- Cabbage
- Carrots
- Cauliflower
- Celery
- Corn
- Leek
- Lettuce
- Eggplant
- Garlic
- Ginger
- Kale
- Onion
- Potatoes
- Parsnips
- Peas
- Pumpkin
- Silver beet
- Spinach

- Spring onions
- Tomatoes
- Turnips
- Zucchini

KNOW WHEN TO CHOOSE ORGANIC!

Bring your "Raw Foods Eating Plan" with you so you know when organic is the better option!

DRIED FRUIT

- Apricots
- Cranberries
- Dates
- Raisins
- Goji berries

FROZEN FRUIT

- Blackberries
- Blueberries

- Mixed berries
- Raspberries

BASICS

- Toilet paper
- Paper towels/napkins
- Re-sealable bags
- Cling wrap
- Aluminium foil
- Trash bags
- Hand soap
- Dish soap
- Detergent
- Stain remover
- Toilet bowl cleaner
- Floor cleaner
- Furniture oil
- Pet food
- Medicine

Protein Powder Alternatives

Why are traditional protein powders a bad health choice for you?

1. **They are very processed.** Consuming chemicals, toxins, and synthetic materials confuses the body. It disrupts hormones and causes the body to search for the missing nutrients, sometimes even leeching them from your body's reserves, such as bones.

2. **They are hard on your body.** The processed materials are hard for your body to break down and your kidneys will have to work extra hard to excrete the toxins. They also often contain whey protein (isolate), soy, and gluten making your liver work extra hard to filter them.

3. **They contain chemical sweeteners.** Ingredients such as fructose, artificial colours, saccharin, and aspartame are commonly present in protein powders. They are toxic and can cause health problems if consumed regularly, and especially so if consumed in large quantities.

4. **They contain heavy metals.** Some protein powders even contain arsenic, lead, cadmium, and mercury.

What are better alternatives to protein powders?

Look for protein powders that contain ingredients that are not artificial or full of chemicals. It's a safe bet that if you can't read the list, it's not a good product option! Instead look for off-the-shelf products that contain the ingredients below, or as an alternative, you can make your own protein smoothies at home yourself.

1. Spirulina
2. Bee pollen (not vegan)
3. Maca
4. Vital Greens
5. Sun Warrior
6. Vega
7. Surthrival Elk Velvet Antler (not vegan, but the animals are free range and slaughter free)

Good Carbs List

USE THE LIST BELOW when menu planning (or grocery shopping)—it provides you with a useful reference for making better carb choices, and includes serving sizes for planning portion amounts.

CARBOHYDRATE	SERVING SIZE
Rice—wild and brown, white, balsamic	1 cup
White potato	1 potato
Sweet potato	1 small potato or 1/2 large potato
Banana	1 banana
Beetroot	1 beetroot
Parsnips	2 parsnips
Celeriac	1 celeriac
Turnip	1 turnip
Nuts or seeds	1 handful
Quinoa	1 cup
Oats, pre-soaked	1 cup
Legumes	1 cup

A

Dietary Fats

○ DIETARY FAT: WHAT'S RIGHT FOR YOU?

Suggested daily fat intake is determined by your body size and weight.

Health authorities recommend you limit your intake of the following types of fats:

- Saturated fat found in meats, butter, cream, or ice cream, and other foods with animal fat
- Trans fat, a man-made fat found in some margarines or packaged goods

Note: *Coconut oil is a saturated fat, but offers many health benefits, so it is an exception to the above rule. Also, clarified butter and eating some animal fat occasionally is okay too.*

HEALTHY DAILY FAT ALLOWANCES

Person weighting between 55 – 80 kg

- 40 to 70 grams of total fat
- 14 grams or less of saturated fat
- 2 grams or less of trans fat

Person weighting between 80 – 100 kg

- 49 to 86 grams of total fat
- 17 grams or less of saturated fat
- 3 grams or less of trans fat

Person weighting 100+ kgs

- 56 to 97 grams of total fat
- 20 grams or less of saturated fat
- 3 grams or less of trans fat.

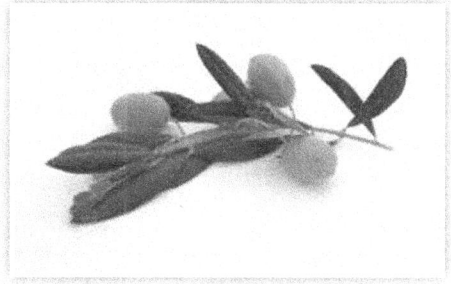

FAT REFERENCE GUIDE per serve

- 1/4 of an avocado
- 6 nuts
- Handful of seeds
- 1 Tbsp olive oil, coconut oil, UDO's, or flax seed oil
- Thumb size pat of butter or ghee
- 1/3 cup almond flour
- 1 cup almond milk
- 2 pieces of organic sugar free chocolate (70% or more dark chocolate)
- 1 Tbsp raw cocoa butter
- 1 Tbsp nut butters (avoid peanut butter)

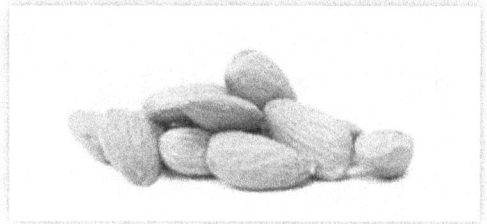

○ THE FACTS ON UNSATURATED FATS

Dietary fat is categorized as saturated or unsaturated. Unsaturated fats—monounsaturated and polyunsaturated—should be the dominant type of fat in a balanced diet, because they reduce the risk of clogged arteries. The items in green font should be avoided.

Monosaturated Fats

While foods tend to contain a mixture of fats, monounsaturated fat is the primary fat found in:

- Recommended: olive, avocado, nuts, such as almonds, cashews, and pistachios
- Avoid: canola oil, sesame oil, peanuts, and peanut butter

Polyunsaturated Fats

- Recommended: flaxseed and flaxseed oil
- Avoid: corn, cottonseed, safflower oil, sunflower seeds and sunflower oil, soybeans and soybean oil, and tub margarine

The Facts on Omega-3 Fats

Seafood is one of your best options for fat. It offers omega-3 fats (DHA or docosahexanoic acid, and EPA, eicosapentanoic acid), which are unsaturated fats considered central to a child's nervous system development, eyesight, and cardiovascular development.

Omega-3 fats can help with reducing blood triglycerides (fats), lowering your risk of blood clots that block the flow of blood to the heart and brain, and help to maintain a normal heart beat.

Seafood contains preformed omega-3 fats, which your body prefers over other fat sources. People can produce DHA and EPA from foods such as walnuts and flax, but studies show that the most efficient sources of omega-3 fats include fatty, cold-water fish, such as salmon, sardines, and tuna.

The Facts on Saturated Fat

Saturated fat has a reputation for developing clogged arteries that restrict, reduce, or even block blood flow, increasing your risk of stroke or heart attack. In fact, saturated fat is more efficient than even dietary cholesterol when it comes to raising blood cholesterol levels.

The most common source of saturated fat is animal meats, and full-fat dairy foods. Animal fats usually supply most of the saturated fat in our diet, and is commonly found even in packaged foods such as crackers and biscuits.

Your body produces all the saturated fat it needs. However, don't worry about completely avoiding all foods with saturated fat, because many of them offer additional benefits such as protein, minerals, vitamins, and more. Limit your saturated fat to less than 7% of all the fat you consume.

The Facts on Trans Fat

Trans fat contributes to clogged arteries just like saturated fat. However, trans fat is a double threat, as it has been linked to breast cancer, colorectal cancer, and others.

Tiny amounts of naturally-occurring trans fat are present in animal proteins and full-fat dairy products; however most trans fat is consumed as a result of hydrogenation of oil, used to extend the shelf life of food. This process converts some of the unsaturated fat to saturated fat.

Thankfully, partially hydrogenated fat (trans fat) has received a lot of attention in the press, drawing attention to this dangerous fat, and the result is that companies are feeling the pressure to remove trans fats from most packaged foods. However, it's still common to find trans fat in stick margarine, fast food, cookies, granola bars, and more. Check product labels and do your best to remain under the daily limit of 2 grams of trans fat per day for adults.

3 Easy Ways to Choose Good Fats...

Below are three easy options for choosing better dietary fats:

1. Choose whole foods made from scratch rather than packaged or processed foods.
2. Use olive or coconut oil or small amounts of butter or ghee for cooking and flavouring foods.
3. Consume an appropriate allowance of good dietary fat at every meal, such as lean meat (RPP plan), legumes, avocado, nuts, and seeds.

Benefits of Zinc

Zinc is a trace element that offers many benefits to your overall health. You should regularly check your zinc levels. Include these foods when your zinc needs a boost!

- Seafood, including crab and oysters (best source)
- Red meat (choose lean)
- Chicken
- Seeds and nuts
- Lamb
- Legumes
- Beans

Average Daily Recommended Amounts for Zinc:

- 8 milligrams for adults
- 11 milligrams if pregnant
- 12 milligrams if breastfeeding

Here is a list of the amazing health and beauty benefits that zinc has to offer you!

- heals wounds
- Boosts testosterone levels
- Builds and repairs muscle
- Produces vitamin A and controls oil production which improves your skin

- Destroys free radicals that are damaging to skin
- Preserves collagen to prevent the development of wrinkles
- Produces keratin which helps you grow healthier nails and hair
- Boosts energy levels naturally
- Activates T lymphocytes that control and regulate immune responses and attack cancer cells
- Assists with proper growth and development during childhood including the ability to learn and memory storage
- Fights impotence
- Prevents osteoporosis in women

RESOURCES:

http://ods.od.nih.gov/factsheets/Zinc-QuickFacts/

http://www.medicalnewstoday.com/articles/263176.php

http://www.webmd.com/vitamins-supplements/ingredientmono-982-ZINC.aspx?activeIngredientId= 982&activeIngredientName=ZINC

Acid vs. Alkaline Foods

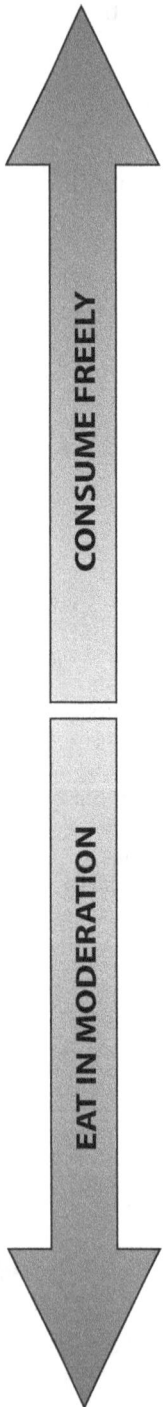

pH			
10.0	Alfalfa grass Artichokes Asparagus Broccoli (raw) Brussels sprouts Carrots	Cauliflower Celery (raw) Collards Cucumbers Ionized water Lemons	Limes Onion Potato skin Spinach (raw) Red cabbage Seaweed
9.0	Alfalfa sprouts Beets Blueberries Dates Eggplant (raw) Figs Grapes	Green beans Greens Herbal/green tea Kiwi Lettuce Mangoes Olive oil	Papayas Pears Peas (raw) Sweet potato Sprouted grains Tangerines
8.0	Almonds Apples Apricots Avocados Bananas Capsicum Cherries	Corn (fresh) Grapefruit Honeydew melon Mushrooms Olives Oranges Peaches	Pineapple Radish Rock melon Strawberries Tomatoes Turnip Wild rice

Optimum pH for human blood is 7.365

pH			
7.0	Butter (unsalted) Cream	Milk (raw cow) Oils (except olive)	Tap water
6.0	Brown rice Cocoa Cold water fish Coconut	Eggs Goat's milk Liver Oysters	Processed juices Salmon Spinach (cooked) Tuna
5.0	Beer Black beans Butter (salted) Canned fruit Corn (cooked)	Garbanzos Lentils Molasses Navy beans Pinto beans	Potatoes w/o skin Rice cakes Sugar Turkey White rice
4.0	Beef Blackberries Bottled/distilled/ purified water Buttermilk	Coffee Cranberries Cream cheese Nuts Popcorn	Prunes Tomato sauce Sweetened fruit juice White bread
3.0	Aspartame Black tea Cheese Chocolate Goat cheese Lack of sleep Lamb	Microwaved foods Overwork Pasta Pastries Pickles Pork Processed foods	Shellfish Soda (pH 2.3) Stress Tobacco smoke Wine Vinegar

Benefits of Apple Cider Vinegar

B RAGG APPLE CIDER VINEGAR (raw, unfiltered, with 'mother') is one of the best products you can store in your pantry. It has many uses that will both promote good health as well as beauty. Avoid taking it neat (undiluted) because it can soften tooth enamel and burn the soft tissue in your mouth, throat, and esophagus. The simple option is to simply dilute 1 - 2 teaspoons of apple cider vinegar and 1 teaspoon of honey in a cup of warm water.

- Anti-bacterial, anti-fungal, and anti-viral
- Soothes sunburnt skin and bug bites
- Removes stain from teeth
- Studies indicate it can aid in weight loss
- Balances your pH values and regulates pH of skin
- Helps detox
- Fights candida (the bacteria associated with yeast infections)
- Hair rinse for shiny hair
- Repels fleas on pets
- Fights allergies, sinus infections, and ear infections
- Soothes sore gums and sore throat
- Used to dissolve kidney stones

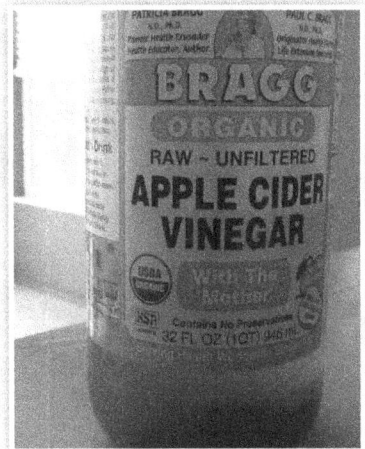

- Lowers high blood pressure and cholesterol
- Gets rid of warts
- Fights nail fungus
- Conditions and detangles hair
- Reduces inflammation, relieves arthritis and gout
- Relieves asthma
- Soothes nausea
- Helps lower glucose levels in diabetes

REFERENCES:

Http://www.mindbodygreen.com/0-5875/15-Reasons-to-Use-Apple-Cider-Vinegar-Every-Day.html

http://thehealthyeatingsite.com/benefits-of-apple-cider-vinegar/

How Sustainable Are You?

A

DO YOU PRACTICE ANY OF THE FOLLOWING OPTIONS FOR LIVING SUSTAINABLY?				
Recycle your paper, plastics, and glass	Yes	☐	No	☐
Grow your own garden (or help with a community garden)	Yes	☐	No	☐
Compost your own soil	Yes	☐	No	☐
Ferment vegies	Yes	☐	No	☐
Grow your own sprouts	Yes	☐	No	☐
Make your own preserves by canning	Yes	☐	No	☐
Store rainwater	Yes	☐	No	☐
Use solar panels for electricity	Yes	☐	No	☐

1) As you grew up, who taught you about ways to live sustainably? (The term "sustainable" may not have been used, of course; just try to think of anything you were taught that made you more self-sufficient.)

2) Do you think your family could benefit from growing your own fruits, vegies, or herbs?

3) Is helping the environment something that is important to you? Why or why not?

4) Do you feel that living sustainably could save your family money? Why or why not?

A

Fermenting Your Vegies

You can ferment your own vegetables by completing the following steps:

1. Shred (or slice very thin) your chosen organic vegies straight into a mason jar, filling it up.

2. Choose one of the following:

A. Juice a batch of organic celery for the brine (this eliminates the need to add sea salt) and pour it into the jar, filling it to the top.

B. Add 1 tsp sea salt and fill the jar with water to the top.

3. *(Optional)* Add a starter culture to the jar, such as kefir grains or a commercial dried starter.

4. Double check to ensure the brine in the jar is *completely* full (no air pocket should be left in the jar).

5. Close the lid with the flat round piece *inverted*, and only loosely close the screw on piece of the lid. Place jar into a bowl, as some of the brine could expand and spill over the sides. Do not close too tightly so that you avoid the top from exploding off!

6. Store in a warm place for 24 - 96 hours. Ideal temperature is 21 degrees Celsius, but don't let it get any warmer than 29 degrees Celsius; if it gets warmer than that, it will kill the healthy microbes. An

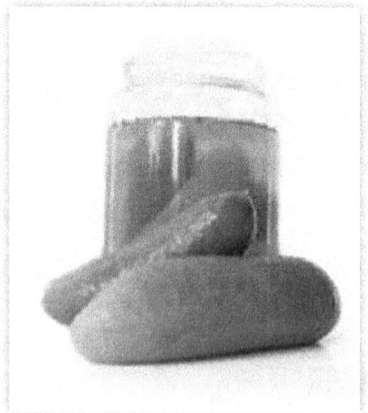

ideal option is to leave the jars in the oven with the *heat off* and the *light bulb on*.

7. After the time has elapsed, tighten the lid up and relocate the jar to the refrigerator to stall the microbe development.

8. After it is chilled, eat and enjoy!

> *When stored, always keep the*
> *fluid level higher than the vegies*
> *so they remain covered...*

A

Making Kombucha

You can brew your own kombucha with the following ingredients:

- 3 liters filtered or purified water
- 1 cup organic white sugar
- 4 organic black tea bags
- kombucha mushroom (keep the liquid that comes with it) or starter culture

---

TIPS:

• You can buy the kombucha 'mushroom' (or SCOBY) online.

• If you take care of your kombucha 'mushroom', then this should be the only time you have to purchase one, since you will reserve some from each batch to make the next one.

Now to make your own kombucha!

1. Get a large pot and boil the water in it.

2. Add the sugar and stir until it is completely dissolved.

3. Add the tea bags. Steep the tea until the water is completely cooled (room temperature).

4. Remove the tea bags and pour the tea into a large glass container.

5. Add the kombucha mushroom (or starter culture), plus the 2/3 cup pre-made kombucha. Cover with a towel or cheesecloth. Move the container to a warm, dark location.

6. Let the kombucha sit for 7 to 10 days. The tea will be ready when the mushroom has grown an extra 'pancake' and the tea is fizzy and sour to taste.

7. Remove the mushroom and store in a closed container in the refrigerator. Transfer the tea to a glass container with a tight-fitting lid, and store that in the refrigerator as well.

8. Chill and enjoy!

TIPS:

• *You can also use fruit teas or green tea bags in your kombucha; just be aware you need 2 of each of those tea bags to replace 1 black tea bag. For example, you could use 2 black tea bags and 4 mango tea bags.*

• *You can also experiment by adding your own freshly squeezed juice to the brewing kombucha after it has been sitting about 5 days.*

Easy Steps to Sprouting

You can grow sprouts in jars right next to your kitchen sink! You will need the following materials:

- wide-mouth jars
- sprouting screen/netting
- bowl for draining
- fresh water
- organic sprouting seeds

TIPS:

• *Always choose organic! If you use seeds that were not harvested for sprouting, they could have chemicals or pesticides on them that will end up in your sprouts.*

• *Roughly 2 ounces of seeds will yield you 1 - 2 lbs of sprouts, and about 8 ounces of beans will give you 1 pound of sprouts.*

• *Go for a temperature between 18C and 25C.*

Grow your own sprouts by completing the following steps:

1. Put 2 to 3 tbsp. of seeds or 3 to 4 tbsp. of beans in a wide mouth jar.

2. Cover with a sprouting screen and screw on the lid.

3. Rinse a couple times, then fill the jar 3/4 full with pure water, room temperature, and soak 6-8 hours or overnight on your benchtop.

4. Drain the soaking water through the screen and rinse 2 or 3 times in cool water.

5. Invert and prop the jar at a downward angle in a bowl (or sink) to drain.

6. For 3 to 5 more days, rinse 2 or 3 times each day in cool water and prop the jar downward in the bowl, just like in step 5.

7. Leave the jar in bright (but not direct) sunlight. The sprouts should be ready to harvest in 3 to 7 days (see note at bottom).

8. Once ready, drain well. Cover the jar with a solid lid, or transfer to a covered container. Refrigerate to store, which slows down the growth of the sprouts and reduces spoilage.

> *Your sprouts are ready to enjoy when they reach the following lengths:*
>
> • *Seed sprouts are ready when they are 2.5 cm - 5 cm long.*
>
> • *Bean sprouts are ready when they are .5 cm - 1 cm long.*
>
> • *Mung beans are ready when they are 2.5 cm - 5 cm long.*

A   What Are My Housecleaning Habits?

If your house is not clean, do you dislike having surprise guests or family over?

_____

_____

_____

How often do you spend cleaning your home each week?

_____

_____

_____

Do you ever go on 'cleaning binges', i.e., hours of rushed cleaning in order to clean up for the arrival of a friend or family member because you felt the house was too dirty for guests? If you have, what does a 'cleaning binge' look like for you?

_____

_____

_____

If you go on 'cleaning binges', what are your stress levels like at that time? Does the atmosphere of the house change?

_____

_____

_____

Do you feel like your house gets too dirty too often?

_____

_____

_____

Do you have a regular cleaning routine? If so, what is it like?

_____

_____

_____

Do you feel like your partner or kids should do more to help keep the house clean?

_____

_____

_____

Do you love the feeling of having a clean home?

_____

_____

_____

MONDAY - FRIDAY
Cleaning Routine

30 minutes daily. Set your timer for each task, grab your Clean-up Caddy and move quickly—you should be able to count this as a workout by the time you are done! You are building habits here, so it is important that you resist the urge to keep cleaning in those rooms after the timer beeps. Leave it where you finish, pick up your stuff, and head to the next task. It's cleaner now than when you started—leave the guilt behind!

Main Bathroom - 5 Minutes

- lean all surfaces (mirror, bench, outside of toilet, weight scale, trash can, and items on bench such as toothbrush holder) using the mirror and surface cleaner and a quality microfiber cloth
- Clean one corner of the tub/shower (switch corner surface each day), starting with the dirtiest corner, using a coarse sponge and appropriate cleaner
- Use plain dish soap or detergent to give the toilet bowl a quick scrub, and then flush

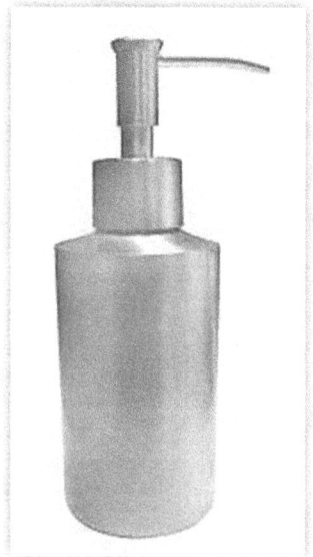

Note: Floors will be cleaned separately; don't worry about them.

Kitchen - 10 Minutes

- Load/unload the dishwasher (or wash the dishes and put away, +10 minutes)
- Wipe down the benchtop and appliance surfaces with soap or another appropriate cleaner for the surface type
- Wipe down backsplash for any grease or smudges
- Sweep
- If the floor is sticky, spot wipe if possible, or decide if you should mop (+10 minutes)

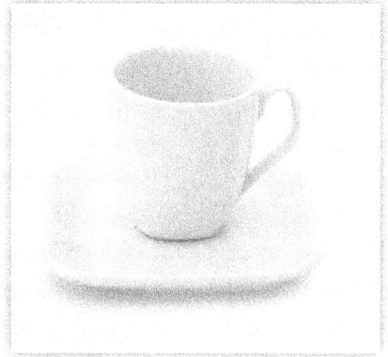

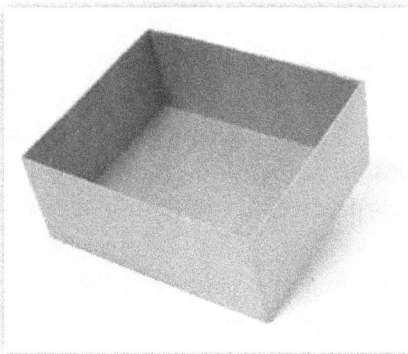

De-Clutter - 5 + 5 Minutes

Grab a box and a trash bag and head to the room that needs the most help with removing clutter: lounge room, family room, kitchen, office, laundry, workout area, game room, etc.

- De-clutter for 5 minutes (Move quickly!)
  - Anything that needs to be thrown away goes into the trash bag
  - Items that need to be donated or relocated go into the box.
- Place the trash bag by the door to throw out
- For the remaining 5 minutes, carry the box through the house:
- Put items away in their 'homes'
  - Anything left in the box that doesn't have a home, put it in another dedicated box marked for donation (Once full, drop it off at a donation center)

Kid's Bedrooms (Daily Inspection for Mum) - 5 Minutes

- Put away toys and clothes
- Wipe up spills (with mum's help at inspection)
- Make bed
- Change sheets (once weekly with mum's help at inspection)

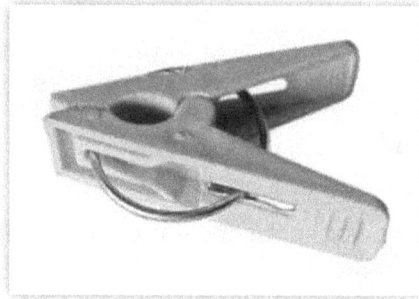

Note: Floors will be cleaned separately; don't worry about them.

Optional: Laundry - 5 Minutes

If your family produces a lot of laundry, wash and dry a load during the week, as appropriate. If you will not have time to fold and put it away the same day, leave the clean, dry clothes in the basket for Sunday. Just make sure it's not the type of load that will matter if it wrinkles (sheets, towels, undies, etc). Ironing more clothes later will just add to your work load. Don't forget to clean out your lint filter!

SATURDAY
Cleaning Routine

It's the weekend—if you've followed your routines, the main bathroom, kitchen, and kid's rooms are basically clean! Let's tackle a few different areas on Saturday.

Floors - 10 Minutes

Sweep and vacuum all floors in the house. Start with the dirtiest room and don't forget to clean the skirting boards! If you don't finish cleaning or sweeping the entire house, stop at 10 minutes—you will start with the dirtiest room next week.

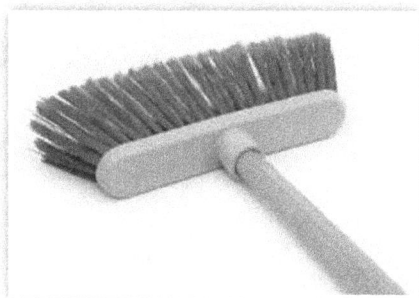

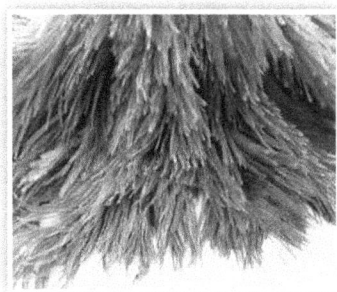

Parent Bedroom - 5 Minutes

- Change the sheets
- Put clothes and clutter away
- Dust

Parent (or Guest) Bathroom - 5 Minutes

- Clean all surfaces (mirror, bench, outside of toilet, weight scale, trash can, and items on bench such as toothbrush holder) using the mirror and surface cleaner and a quality microfiber cloth

- Clean one corner of the tub/shower (switch corner surface each day), starting with the dirtiest corner, using a coarse sponge and appropriate cleaner

- Use plain dish soap or detergent to give the toilet bowl a quick scrub, and then flush

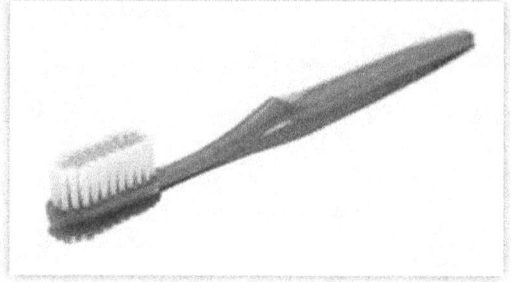

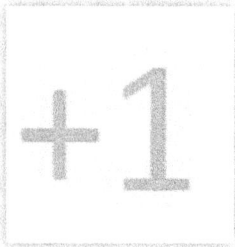

One Extra Room - 10 Minutes

Pick one extra room in the house to dust and de-clutter, as needed.

Now *go enjoy your day*, no matter what your house looks like!

SUNDAY
Cleaning Routine

Laundry - Time Varies by Family Size

- Wash, fold, and put away

Replenish & Refresh - 5 Minutes

- Change towels and washcloths for kitchen and all bathrooms
- Put out toilet paper rolls in all bathrooms

Pick One Bonus Activity - 15 Minutes

Pick a room for extra cleaning and de-cluttering/organizing!

- Clean the inside and top of fridge
- Sweep the entrance and back deck
- Organize a shelf or cabinet contents
- Wipe cabinet doors
- Iron clothes
- Clean out the car and check oil levels
- Clean blinds
- Clean windows
- Extra vacuuming time
- Weed the garden
- Clean out dryer exhaust

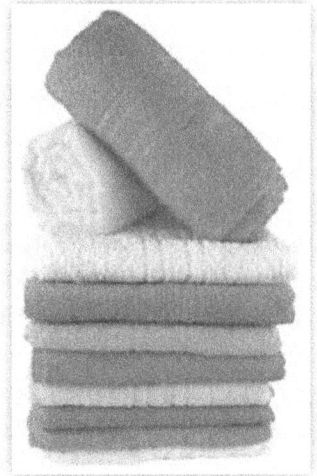

- Organize the garage
- Dust ceiling fans
- Dust ceilings, corners, and walls
- Home maintenance

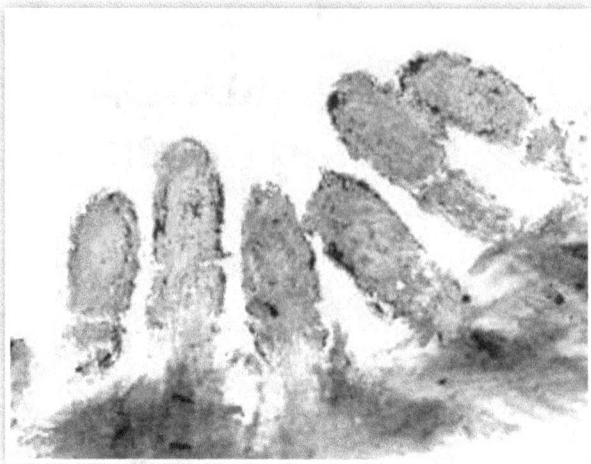

Learn to clean and LET GO!

Once you have given your 30 minutes, stop, put your cleaning cloths away to wash, leave your caddy in place for the next day, and GO!

You succeeded!

6 MONTH DEEP
Cleaning Routine

Make this fun! Turn on fun music, wear something comfortable, and get the kids to help. Make food the night before, and if your kids are younger, "picnic" inside on a blanket for lunch to make it unique, or picnic in the back yard (if weather permits). Attack the list below row by row, or go room by room.

LOCATION	CLEANING
All rooms	Clean baseboards with vinegar Dust top of doors, frames, and window sills using water or vinegar Dust walls and corners for cobwebs Wipe smudges off of switch plates and power point covers Clean mirrors Remove blinds and wash outside (if you don't clean them regularly) Clean inside of windows Change batteries in smoke detectors Once a year - have rugs and carpets cleaned
Kitchen	Clean under/around/on top of appliances Wipe grease from underside or top of vent hood, and clean filters Clean top of cabinets (if they don't extend to ceiling height) Wipe front of cabinets Clean out inside of cabinets and organize Clean inside of oven Organize under sink Seal benchtops (if applicable) Wipe down canisters or other items on benchtop

LOCATION	CLEANING
Bedrooms	Flip mattresses Clean and vacuum under beds Organize and vacuum/sweep closets Clean out inside of drawers and organize Wash mattress pad Clean shelves Wash or dry clean curtains
Bathrooms	Clean out medicine cabinets Wipe front and top of cabinets Clean out inside of vanity and organize Wipe weight scale Clean shower door Soak bathtub toys in sink with apple cider vinegar, then scrub sink
Lounge / Family Room / Game Room	Dust plants (or take outside and lightly rinse) and fertilize Clean and vacuum under furniture Clean under the lounge cushions Spot treat stains on fabrics / Once clean and dry, apply ScotchgardTM Throw out magazines
Office	Clean out inside of desk drawers and organize Dust bookshelves Clean out paperwork, file, and throw away old receipts (office) Wipe down computer and computer screen with lightly damp microfiber cloth Make quick list of supplies needed (stamps, pens, paper clips, etc.)

LOCATION	CLEANING
Outside	Clean outside of windows Knock down spider webs and wasp nests Cut back dead plants and throw into the compost pile Wash driveway, sidewalks Organize garage cabinets Organize outside freezer and make note of contents
Car	Vacuum floor and under seats Wipe dashboard and interior surfaces with suitable cleaner Wash, then wax and wipe outside Check engine fluids and condition of wipers Check spare tire condition Ensure safety kit (jumper cables, reflectors, etc.) is in the boot

A

Household Cleaning Recipes

The primary ingredients needed are white vinegar, baking soda, borax (or washing soap), liquid vegie soap (or castile soap, such as Dr. Bronner's) and hydrogen peroxide. For scent, tea tree oil is a good choice and also has anti-bacterial properties. You can find liquid vegie soap online or in natural living stores. Another option is to purchase Sal Suds by Dr. Bonner's for overall cleaning.

Basic Surface and Glass Cleaner

Mix 4 parts water to 1 part white vinegar and water in a spray bottle.

Household Surface Grime Cleaner (with Soap)

- 1 part liquid vegie soap
- 3 parts borax or baking soda
- Add a few drops tea tree oil

Combine. Pour into spray bottle and *add hot water* to the desired consistency. Shake to mix. Make as needed.

Scrubbing Cleaner

3 parts baking soda or borax to 1 part liquid vegie soap or water. Mix. If you need to increase abrasiveness, add more baking soda/borax. Add a few drops of tea tree oil if storing in closed container.

Clothing Detergent

- 1/4 to 1/3 cup of Dr. Bronner's castile soap (or read label for Sal Suds)

- dash of baking soda or washing soap
- 1/2 cup vinegar to rinse cycle

Divide in half for front loading, high-efficiency washers. Plus, less soap is fine for lightly soiled clothes.

Bleaching Alternative for Clothes

¼ cup hydrogen peroxide or vinegar added to wash.

Dishwasher Detergent

- 2 cups borax or baking soda
- 1/2 cup sea salt
- 1/4 cup citric acid

Combine and store in airtight container. Use 1 - 2 tbsp. per load. Put vinegar in rinsing reservoir.

Drain Cleaner

Pour the following items down the drain, in order.

1. 1 cup baking soda
2. 1 cup white vinegar
3. Let soak for a few minutes
4. Pour very hot or boiling water down drain.

Toilet Bowl Cleaner

- ½ cup baking soda
- 1 cup white vinegar
- 1 tsp tea tree oil

Combine in spray bottle, spray inside bowl, on seat, lid, etc. Let it sit for a few minutes. Then add a little extra baking soda to the inside of the bowl and scrub with a toilet brush.

You will only need to use this occasionally because you will be cleaning your toilets frequently. Normally you can scrub with just the brush, or if you want extra deodorizing, spray the inside of the bowl with vinegar, scrub, and flush to rinse.

Surface Mold Killer

- Fill a spray bottle container with enough hot water to do the job
- For every cup in the container add about 25 drops of tea tree oil

Spray on the surface with mold, allow to sit for a few minutes, and pat dry with a paper towel. For a stronger option, replace the tea tree oil with 1 part hydrogen peroxide.

Carpet Stains

1. Combine equal parts vinegar and baking soda (mix right before using as it froths up)
2. Work into the carpet stain using a brush with bristles (even an old toothbrush would work)
3. Allow to dry completely
4. Vacuum

Identify Your Unhealthy Lifestyle Habits

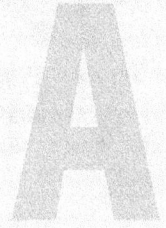

A

This questionnaire is divided into categories. In each section, read the question and then place a mark in the column to the right that best matches your answer. If any questions do not apply to you, then place the mark in the N/A column.

QUESTIONS	DAILY	WEEKLY	SOMETIMES	NO	N/A
About You					
Do you spend time in prayer or meditation?					
Do you keep a journal?					
Do you express gratefulness for your life when talking to others?					
Do you have hobbies you practice?					
Do you spend time outdoors?					
Do you often feel stressed?					
Do you take care of your health?					
Do you treat yourself to special things (clothes, manicure, etc.)?					

QUESTIONS	DAILY	WEEKLY	SOMETIMES	NO	N/A
Relationship with Partner					
Do you make time for your spouse or significant other?					
Do you have an active sex life?					
Do you keep a regular date night?					
Do you spend any time away from the kids? (Holidays, meeting for lunch, etc.)					
Do you express appreciation for your spouse?					
Do you feel your spouse expresses appreciation for you?					
Are you able to communicate concerns with each other?					

QUESTIONS	DAILY	WEEKLY	SOMETIMES	NO	N/A
Relationship with Kids					
How old are your kids? _____					
Do you make time for your kid's activities?					
Do you tell others how proud you are of your kid's accomplishments?					
Do you spend time alone with each of your kids?					
Do you tell your kids that you love each one as a unique and special person?					

Food For Health

QUESTIONS	DAILY	WEEKLY	SOMETIMES	NO	N/A
Life Skills					
Have you taught your kids any of the following life skills? (If not age appropriate choose N/A)	**Yes**	**No**	**N/A**		
Laundry					
Ironing					
Gardening/landscaping					
Cooking/baking/menu planning					
Balance a chequebook					
Mend a hem or button					
Basic car repairs					
Mow the lawn					
Make the bed					
Volunteering					

SCORING

- Daily receives +4 points
- Weekly receives +3 points
- Sometimes receives +2 points
- No deducts -1 point
- Yes receives +3 points
- No deducts -1 point
- N/A responses are neutral (0 points)

Add up the total for all columns; then add together.

Daily	_____	Yes	_____
Weekly	_____	No	_____
Sometimes	_____	N/A	_____
No	_____	**Overall Total**	_____

RESULTS

0 - 40 = Nurturing yourself and the relationships in your life will offer good improvement for your health.

41 - 70 = Not too bad. You try to reach out, but you're struggling with time or some other barrier.

71 - 110 = You put consistent effort into taking care of yourself and managing your relationships.

111+ = You are a master at managing your health and maintaining the relationships in your life! Congrats!

Skincare Recipes

Everybody needs a little pampering occasionally! Not only is it good for you body, it can be mentally and emotionally healthy to indulge in a favorite beauty routine. The skincare recipes below are good for your body, your mind, your heart—and your purse! Only use 1 treatment per day; do not combine treatments.

Clay Mask Exfoliation

Buy white or green clay from a natural living store. Mix 1 tbsp. clay with:

- cream for dry skin
- milk for normal skin
- water for oily skin

Wash face first, then pat dry. Use enough liquid to make the clay easily spreadable. Mix in a bowl and spread on face. Leave until dry and then wash off and pat your face dry. Follow with a healthy face moisturizer.

Poor Reduction Mask

- 1/2 cup freshly mashed papaya
- 2 tsp raw pineapple juice

Wash face first, then pat dry. Mix until a smooth paste is formed. Spread on face and lie down for 15 - 20 minutes with a towel wrapped around your face, as the mix is pretty runny. It is normal for the mask to feel tingly. Rinse after no more than 20 minutes. Follow with a healthy face moisturizer.

Body Scrub

- Pour 1/2 cup cane sugar (or sea salt) in a sealable jar

- Enough olive oil or jojoba oil to cover the sugar, plus an extra 1 centimeter
- Add a few drops of your favorite essential oil

After combining, put the airtight lid on the container. Leave next to the tub. Pour out or use a wooden or stainless steel spoon to scoop some out. Moisten your body first, then apply the scrub. Rub gently until exfoliated, then rinse. Follow with a health body moisturizer.

Nighttime Moisturizer for the Eyelids

- 1/4 tsp of olive oil or jojoba oil

Do not apply directly on eye. Wash face first, then pat dry. Dip fingers in oil and pat gently on eyelid and under eyes, avoiding the eye duct area. Follow with a healthy face moisturizer for the rest of your face.

Congestion Relief

Help for when a cold or lung congestion has you down! Note: Always see your doctor for health concerns.

- 3 cups distilled water
- 2 drops each: peppermint, eucalyptus (E. radiate), and juniper essential oils

Boil the water. Let sit for 1 minute with lid on. Add essential oil drops. Pour into bowl that can handle hot water. Drape a towel over your head and lean over bowl, with eyes closed, about 10 - 12 inches from bowl. Breath deeply and relax for 10 minutes.

Identify Your Unhealthy Financial Habits

A

This worksheet is divided into categories. In each section, read the question and then place a mark in the column to the right that best matches your answer. If any questions do not apply to you, then place the mark in the N/A column.

QUESTIONS	YES	NO	N/A
Are you aware of how much money comes into your home every month?			
Are you aware of how much your bills cost you each month?			
Do you pay off all your credit card balances every month, or at least every 2 months?			
Do you have only one mortgage on your home?			
Can you afford to properly insure your home and car?			
Do you spend less than one quarter of your monthly income on your mortgage?			
Is your income enough to sustain the family (i.e., you do not have to borrow from family or get a loan)?			
Are you paying bills on time and therefore able to avoid paying late charges, overdraft fees, and surcharges?			
Are your relationships suffering because of finances?			
Are you living within your means?			
Are you putting money into savings?			
Are you putting money towards retirement?			

Add up your No responses.

1 - 3 = Not too bad. You have issues to address, but with a few small changes, you'll be in good shape.

3+ = You have financial issues that need to be addressed immediately. Big changes and even sacrifices may be required to correct your financial woes.

Your Family Budget

Pull out your recent bills, pay stubs, receipts, and bank statements, then complete the fields below. Do not include one-time payments—just the typical or average expenses and income.

INCOME		Child Support	
Monthly Income	_____	Other Income / Deposits	_____
Alimony	_____	TOTAL INCOME	_____

FIXED EXPENSES		Alimony/Child Support	
1st Mortgage or Rental	_____	Payment	_____
2nd Mortgage or Rental	_____	Home Phone	_____
Home or Rental Insurance	_____	Mobile Phone	_____
Home Association Dues	_____	Internet	_____
Real Estate Taxes	_____	Cable	_____
1st Car Payment	_____	Life Insurance	_____
2nd Car Payment	_____	Private Health Insurance	_____
Car Insurance	_____	Disability Insurance	_____
Rego Tags	_____	Child Care	_____
Electricity	_____	Tuition	_____
Gas	_____	Student Loans	_____
Water	_____	Subscriptions or Dues	_____
Rubbish	_____	Miscellaneous	_____
		TOTAL FIXED EXPENSES	_____

VARIABLE EXPENSES		SAVINGS	
Food	_____	Savings Account	_____
Petrol	_____	401K/Stock	_____
Clothing	_____	Retirement	_____
Vehicle Repairs	_____	TOTAL SAVINGS	_____
Home Repairs	_____		
Medication	_____		
Pet Food	_____	TOTALS	
Personal Care/Hygiene	_____	Total Income	_____
Miscellaneous	_____	Total Fixed Expenses	_____
TOTAL VARIABLE		Total Variable Expenses	_____
EXPENSES	_____	Total Savings	_____
		TOTAL OVER/UNDER	_____

Grocery Store Comparison Chart

A

FOOD ITEMS	GREEN GROCER	HEALTH FOOD SHOP	WOOL WORTHS	COLES	OTHER/ ONLINE
SWEETNERS	$	$	$	$	$
Agave syrup					
Honey (raw)					
Maple syrup (organic)					
Dark chocolate					
Vanilla extract (gluten free)					
OILS	$	$	$	$	$
Flaxseed oil					
Grapeseed oil					
Olive oil					
Coconut oil (organic)					
Sesame oil					
UDO's oil					
Safflower oil					
Cacao butter					
VINEGARS	$	$	$	$	$
Apple cider vinegar					
Balsamic Vinegar					
Rice wine vinegar					

FOOD ITEMS	GREEN GROCER	HEALTH FOOD SHOP	WOOL WORTHS	COLES	OTHER/ ONLINE
SEEDS	$	$	$	$	$
Chia					
Linseeds					
Poppy seeds					
Pumpkin/Pepitas					
Sesame seeds					
Sunflower seeds					
Quinoa – seeds					
Quinoa – puffed					
Tahina					
Wholegrain mustard/ Dijon					
POWDERS	$	$	$	$	$
Acai					
Cacao powder					
Green Qi/Super Greens					
Maca					
Pea protein					
Raw carob powder					
Sea powder/Kelp					
Spirulina					
SPICES	$	$	$	$	$
Black pepper					
Caraway seeds					
Celtic sea salt					
Cinnamon					
Curry					
Paprika					
Massel stock – beef, chicken, vegie					
Nama shoyu/Tamari					

FOOD ITEMS	GREEN GROCER	HEALTH FOOD SHOP	WOOL WORTHS	COLES	OTHER/ ONLINE
FLOURS	$	$	$	$	$
Almond meal					
Arrowroot					
Baking powder – gluten free					
Coconut – desiccated, shredded					
Coconut flour					
GRAINS AND LEGUMES	$	$	$	$	$
Corn chips/Beetroot corn					
Lentils					
Beans\					
Nori sheets					
Oats					
Rice – black					
Rice – brown					
Rice – white					
Rice cakes					
Rice paper					
DAIRY	$	$	$	$	$
Cheese					
Cream					
Yoghurt – coconut					
MEAT / PROTEIN	$	$	$	$	$
Bacon (nitrate free)					
Beef					
Chicken–breast, thighs, etc.					
Seafood (fish/prawns)					
Goat					
Kabana					
Kangaroo					

FOOD ITEMS	GREEN GROCER	HEALTH FOOD SHOP	WOOL WORTHS	COLES	OTHER/ ONLINE
MEAT / PROTEIN	$	$	$	$	$
Lamb					
Marrow bones–stock/dog					
Mince–beef, chicken, pork					
Pork					
Sausages – gluten free					
Tinned fish – salmon, tuna					
NUTS	$	$	$	$	$
Almond					
Brazil					
Cashew					
Hazelnut					
Pine nuts					
Pistachio					
Walnut					
SALAD	$	$	$	$	$
Avocado					
Celery					
Lettuce					
Spring onions					
Tomatoes-cherry					
Tomatoes- large					
Ginger					
FRUIT	$	$	$	$	$
Bananas					
Apples – red, green					
Kiwi					
Grapes					
Honey dew melon					
Oranges/Mandarin					
Mango					

Food For Health
TURNING THE FOOD PYRAMID ON ITS HEAD

FOOD ITEMS	GREEN GROCER	HEALTH FOOD SHOP	WOOL WORTHS	COLES	OTHER/ ONLINE
FRUIT	$	$	$	$	$
Passion fruit					
Pears					
Pineapple					
Rock melon					
Strawberries					
Watermelon					
VEGETABLES	$	$	$	$	$
Asparagus					
Beans					
Beetroot					
Broccoli					
Brown onions					
Brussels sprouts					
Carrots					
Cauliflower					
Coconut – whole "green"					
Corn					
Leek					
Egg plant					
Garlic					
Green cabbage					
Kale					
Potatoes					
Peas					
Red onions					
Pumpkin					
Red cabbage					
Spinach					
Silver beet					
Zucchini					

FOOD ITEMS	GREEN GROCER	HEALTH FOOD SHOP	WOOL WORTHS	COLES	OTHER/ ONLINE
DRIED FRUIT	$	$	$	$	$
Apricots					
Cranberries					
Dates					
Raisins					
Goji berries					
FROZEN FRUIT	$	$	$	$	$
Blueberries					
Mixed berries					
Raspberries					
Blackberries					
CLEANING SUPPLIES	$	$	$	$	$
Washing powder					
Baking soda					
White vinegar					
Liquid vegie soap					
Borax					
Sal Suds					
Citric acid					
Hydrogen peroxide					
Tea tree oil					
Spray bottles					
MISCELLANEOUS	$	$	$	$	$
Dog/cat/chook food					
Toilet paper					
Paper towels/Napkins					
Re-sealable bags					
Garbage bags					
Aluminium foil					
Cling wrap					

FOOD ITEMS	GREEN GROCER	HEALTH FOOD SHOP	WOOL WORTHS	COLES	OTHER/ ONLINE
MISCELLANEOUS	$	$	$	$	$
Hand soap					
Dish soap					
Detergent					
Furniture polish					
Medicine					
Other:					

Daily 'To Do' List

Date: _____   Su M T W Th F Sa

Must Do

- ☐ _____
- ☐ _____

To Do

- ☐ _____
- ☐ _____
- ☐ _____
- ☐ _____
- ☐ _____
- ☐ _____
- ☐ _____
- ☐ _____

Drink Your Water

1   2   3   4   5   6   7   8

Meals

- ☐ _____
- ☐ _____

Today' s Routines

- ☐ _____
- ☐ _____
- ☐ _____
- ☐ _____
- ☐ _____

Notes

_____

_____

_____

_____

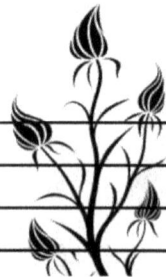

APPENDIX B

B

9 Day 'Get Started' Meal Plan

SHOPPING LIST

- 1 BBQ chicken, shredded (freeze until use)
- 1 kg lean mince
- lamb
- 4 cans sandwich tuna
- 1 large can salmon or tuna in spring water
- 4 slices ham
- 3 dozen eggs
- 1 tomato
- 1 red onion
- 8 apples
- 4 mandarins
- 1 bunch kale
- 2 bananas
- 2 carrots
- 8 dates
- 1 head cos lettuce
- 1 head broccoli
- 1 head cabbage
- 2 avocados
- 3 cucumbers
- 3 - 4 zucchinis
- 2 sweet potatoes
- 1 capsicum
- 1 beetroot
- 1 pumpkin
- 2 onions
- 1 bunch basil
- Mixed greens
- Nori sheets
- 1 (800 ml) can coconut water
- 2 (400 ml) cans coconut milk
- 1 jar red curry paste
- 1 container curry powder
- 1 jar stock cubes, gluten free
- 1 jar coconut oil
- 1 container Super Greens
- 3 cups quinoa
- 1 small bag brazil nuts
- 1 small bag pepitas seeds
- 1 small bag sunflower seeds

- 1 clove garlic
- 1 jar honey
- 1 jar soy sauce, gluten free
- parmesan cheese

EASY SPANISH OMELETTE (Serves 1)

- 2 eggs
- 1 tbsp. butter
- 1 tomato, diced
- 1/4 red onion, diced
- 2 mushrooms, diced or sliced
- basil leaves, torn

Whisk eggs in bowl. Heat tbsp of butter in pan. Thinly spread egg mix in pan, and on one half of egg add: diced tomato, torn basil leaves, red onion, and mushrooms. Fold egg over when cooked and slide onto plate.

GREEN SMOOTHIE (Serves 1)

- 200 ml coconut water
- handful ice
- handful kale
- 1/2 frozen banana
- handful frozen berries
- 2 dates or spoon of honey
- scoop of Super Greens

Combine and blend in blender.

BREKKY MUFFINS (Approx. 6 muffins)

- 6 eggs

- Leftover cooked mince from previous night
- optional: capsicum, diced
- optional: zucchini, diced
- optional: chopped herbs

Whisk eggs. Spoon heaped tbsp. mince into greased muffin tin. Optional add vegies over mince, pour egg over and sprinkle herbs on top, if desired. Bake on 180 for 25 - 30 minutes.

TUNA WRAPS / HAM WRAPS (Serves 1)

- 1 serve sandwich tuna OR ham
- 2 large cos lettuce leaves
- 1 tbsp. sunflower seeds
- 1/2 avocado
- 1/2 cucumber sliced

(Put together when ready to eat.) Place lettuce leaves on plate. Add tuna or ham. Top with avocado, cucumber, and seeds. Wrap and eat fresh.

SUSHI (Serves 1)

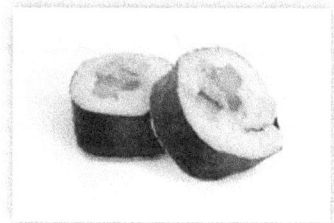

- 1/4 head cauliflower, grated

- 1 Nori sheet
- 1 serve BBQ chicken
- 2 slices avocado

Microwave grated cauliflower for 3 minutes and spoon onto Nori sheet. Add shredded chicken, avocado, and roll up. Cut in half and serve.

CHICKEN SALAD (Serves 1)

- 1 serving BBQ chicken
- Greens
- Pumpkin or sunflower seeds
- Vegies of choice, diced or chopped
- Olive oil, drizzling
- Lemon, squeeze

Mix the BBQ chicken with an assortment of greens. Sprinkle with pepitas or sunflower seeds. Add vegies of choice, drizzle with olive oil and a squeeze of lemon.

QUINOA CURRY (Serves 2)

- 1 cup quinoa
- 1 (400ml) can coconut milk
- 1/2 cup vegetable broth (or water)
- 1 1/2 tbsp. red curry paste
- 2 tbsp. honey
- Optional: 1 tbsp. Sriracha sauce (spicy!)
- 1 tsp. coconut oil
- 1 clove garlic, minced
- 3 cups colorful veggies (onions, carrots, red capsicum, broccoli, etc)
- Fresh basil and/or cilantro (coriander)

Mix quinoa, coconut milk, vegetable broth, red curry paste, honey, and Sriracha sauce (if using) in a medium saucepan and bring to boil. Lower heat to lowest setting. Cover saucepan and simmer until quinoa is ready (about 15 minutes).

While quinoa is cooking, heat oil over medium heat and stir fry the garlic and veggies. Mix veggies with quinoa and serve. Garnish with fresh basil/cilantro.

CHOW MEIN (Serves 2)

- 500 grams mince (or if cooking extra for brekky muffins the next morning, make 1 kg)
- 1 onion, diced
- coconut oil or butter, knob
- 2 tbsp. curry powder
- 1 tbsp. soy sauce, gluten free
- 1 cup quinoa
- 1 1/2 cups stock
- 1/2 cabbage
- 1 carrot, grated (+ other vegies as desired)

Brown mince in pan with diced onion in a knob of coconut oil or butter. Add curry powder, soy cauce. Once browned, reserve half for brekky muffins, if you made the 1 kg. Add quinoa, stock, cabbage, carrot and other vegies. Put lid on and simmer for 15 - 20 minutes, stirring occasionally.

TUNA BAKE (Serves 2)

- 8 eggs
- 1 can corn, drained
- 1 can tuna in spring water
- 1 bunch spring onions
- fresh basil
- 3 zucchinis sliced thin
- Parmesan cheese

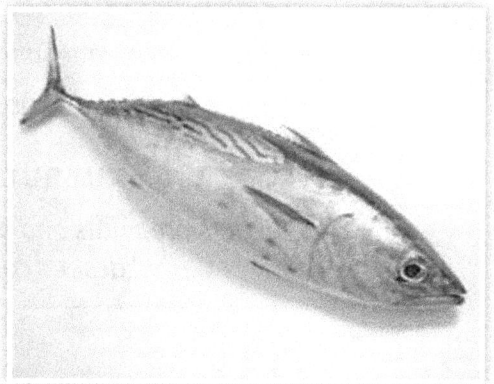

Layer zucchini, corn, onion, and tuna, then pour over egg mixture. Add basil to taste. Sprinkle with parmesan cheese. Bake in oven on 180 for 30 minutes or until cooked.

Food For Health

ROAST LAMB AND VEGIES (Serves 2)

- Combine lamb and vegies of choice in glass

ROAST VEGETABLE SOUP (Varies)

- Use left over roast vegetables. Blend with vegetable stock, add coconut milk and curry to taste, and serve.

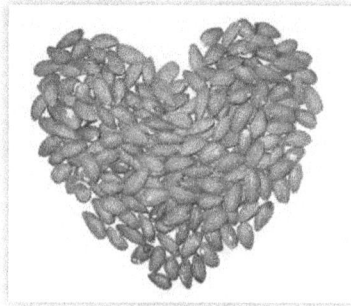

ACTIVATED ALMONDS

NUT MILK:

1. Soak 1 cup almonds overnight

2. Squeeze in batches, reserve water

3. Add to blender and blitz with nuts

4. And 3 cups water

NUT BUTTER:

Blend activated nuts and oil with a pinch of salt until desired consistency.

Breakfast

COCONUT YOGURT

- 1 green coconut
- 2 probiotics
- Glass jar

Open coconut, reserve flesh, add coconut water to your liking, blitz till turned to a thick coconut cream, add 2 probiotics per large jar, screw lid on tightly and leave on the bench for 12 hours. Relocate to fridge for 1 - 2 days and enjoy. Or dehydrate on 41C in jar, store in fridge, chill, and enjoy.

GRANOLA

- Almonds – pre soaked & crushed
- Sunflower seeds
- Pumpkin seeds
- Shredded coconut
- Cranberries
- Raisins
- Coconut oil
- Agave syrup
- Oats or puffed quinoa

Instructions:

1. Set oven 180 deg.
2. Line baking tray.
3. Place dry ingredients on tray.
4. Drizzle with coconut oil and syrup.
5. Bake for 20 minutes.
6. Store in an airtight jar.

GREEN PANCAKES

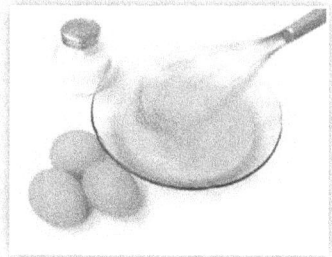

- ½ cup shredded coconut
- ½ cup oats
- 2 cups organic fresh spinach

- 1 tbsp pea protein
- 2 eggs
- 1/8 tsp baking powder

Serve with:

- nut butter and honey
- maple syrup and banana
- Berry sauce:
- frozen berries

- 1 tbsp coconut flour
- 2 tbsp maple syrup

Instructions:

1. Simmer on low till thickens slightly.
2. Blend in food processor.
3. Pan fry as normal.

Main Meals

BAKED MEATBALLS

- 1kg of your choice of mince
- 1 clove garlic, minced
- ½ tbsp salt
- 1 tbsp caraway seeds
- 1 tbsp ground paprika
- 1 tbsp ground black pepper
- 1 tbsp grainy mustard
- 1 cup fresh parsley leaves, minced (¼ cup)
- 1 large egg

Instructions:

1. Preheat oven 100 deg.
2. Cover a large baking tray with baking paper/ aluminium foil.
3. In a large bowl, mix spices and egg with a fork/whisk until combined and add mince and mix until all ingredients are incorporated.
4. Moisten your hands with water and shake to remove excess.
5. Measure a level tbsp of mince and roll into a ball between your palms.
6. Place on tray 1 ½ inches apart and bake for 20 - 25 min until brown and cooked through.

COCONUT LAKSA

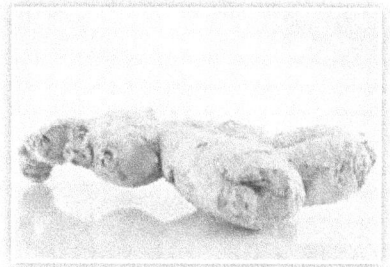

- Combine coconut water, lemon grass, ginger, raw

zucchini noodles, chilli, coriander, and let sit for a few hours. Serve.

STIR FRY

- Stir fry vegies in coconut oil and sesame seeds.

SUSHI

- Cauliflower 'Rice' – grate, steam, season with parsley/herb, cool

Filling:

- Capsicum
- Avocado
- Tomato
- Alfalfa
- Mung beans
- Celery
- Salmon
- Chicken

Spread rice on Nori sheets. Add any desired filling (be creative). Roll and serve.

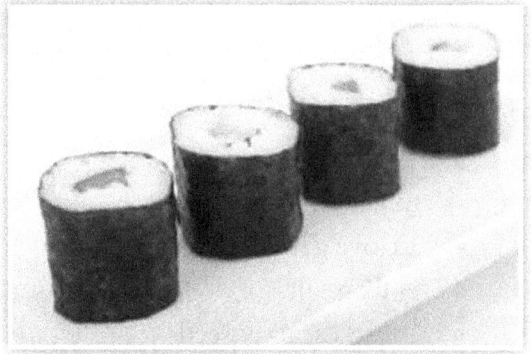

Salads

APPLE CARROT BEETROOT SALAD

Grate all ingredients and serve.

ASIAN SALAD

- wombok, sliced
- 2 sheets Nori, shredded
- serving crushed cashews

Combine. Dress with 2 tbsp. Udo's oil plus 1 tbsp. palm sugar, grated.

CARROT AND RAISIN SALAD

- Grated carrot
- Raisins

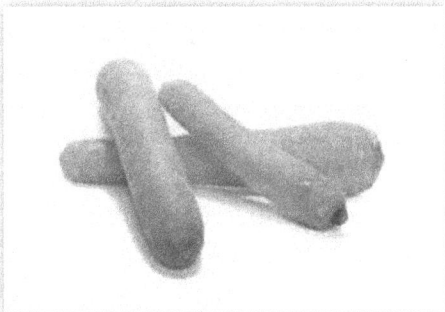

Combine. Dress with Udo's oil and apple cider vinegar.

CAULIFLOWER AND ORANGE SALAD

- cauliflower, grated
- 3 spring onions, sliced
- 2 oranges, segmented
- handful of raisins

Dress with juice from one orange, 1 tbsp. Udo's oil and 2 tbsp. apple cider vinegar.

GREEN SALAD

- 2 Lebanese cucumbers, cubed
- 10 black olives
- 2 tomatoes, chopped
- ½ onion
- fresh parsley
- 1 - 2 tbsp. olive oil
- Add salt to taste

Combine and serve.

GREEN SALAD

- bag of greens
- toss in Udo's olive oil
- fresh/dried oregano
- 1 tbsp. apple cider vinegar

Combine and serve.

KALE SALAD

- Tear and de-stem kale.
- Sprinkle with salt and lemon juice.
- Stir through diced tomatoes.

LEBANESE TOMATO AND AVOCADO SALAD

- 3 tomatoes, skinned and diced
- 2 avocados, chopped
- 3 Lebanese cucumbers, diced

Dress with juice from 2 lemons, 2 tbsp. Udo's oil, and salt to taste.

MUSHROOM SALAD

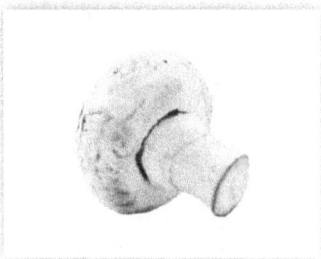

- 500 grams mushrooms, sliced

- bunch of sprint onions, sliced
- 1 clove garlic, grated
- 2 tbsp. Udo's oil

Combine and serve.

RAINBOW COLESLAW

- cabbage
- carrot
- capsicum
- apple
- 1/4 onion

Shred all vegies and steam. Serve.

SIMPLE COLESLAW

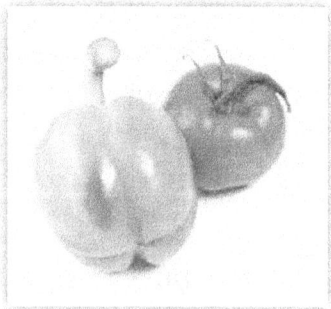

- Shred cabbage and grate carrot.

SPINACH PUMPKIN SALAD

- roast pumpkin cubes
- stir into bag of baby spinach
- 1/2 cup toasted pine nuts
- 1 tbsp. maple syrup
- 2 tbsp. olive oil

Combine pumpkin and spinach. Dress with pine nuts, maple syrup, and olive oil.

TOMATO SALAD

- 4 tomatoes, diced
- 1/4 cup olive oil
- salt
- dried oregano

Combine and leave to sit for 10 minutes. Serve fresh.

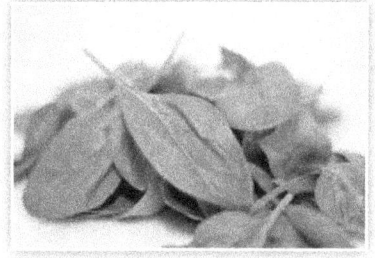

B

Sides

BROCCOLI TABOULI

- broccoli head, grated
- handful of parsley
- handful semi-dried tomatoes, or fresh

Combine and serve. Also nice with pumpkin and sunflower kernels.

CAULIFLOWER 'RICE'

Grate cauliflower. Heat in pot with a few tbsp. water and Massel brand stock cubes. Stir for a few minutes and serve.

FENNEL

Slice thick and sprinkle with salt and a squeeze of lemon juice. Leave for 10 minutes. Serve.

GUACAMOLE

- 1 avocado, mashed
- ½ red onion
- 1 clove garlic
- juice from 1 lemon

Combine and serve fresh.

KALE CHIPS

- Use about 1 bunch of kale. Tear the leaves off the thick stems into bite size pieces. Spread out on cookie sheets.
- Drizzle with about 2 tsp of olive oil or (even better) coconut oil.
- Sprinkle with Parmesan, or your seasonings of choice. Plus a sprinkle of salt.
- Preheat oven to about 190 c . Bake for about 15 minutes, until edges are brown and kale is crispy when moved in pan.

PARSNIP 'RICE'

- Grate parsnips. Season with sesame oil tamari and spring onion, and serve.

ROASTED VEGIES

- Roast vegies in garlic, ghee, and rosemary. Bake 180 degrees until cooked.

SPICY CARROT DIP

- 4 medium carrots steamed
- 1 tsp each of ground cumin, coriander and curry powder
- 1 1/2 cups tinned chickpeas rinsed and drained
- Pinch sea salt
- 1/2 cup tahini
- Juice and zest of 1 orange
- 2 large organic rice cakes per meal
- Optional: add any extra vegetables to topping

Instructions:

1. Puree all ingredients in a food processor, and season with sea salt and pepper to taste.
2. Spread thickly on large rice cakes and add any other vegetable topping you like.

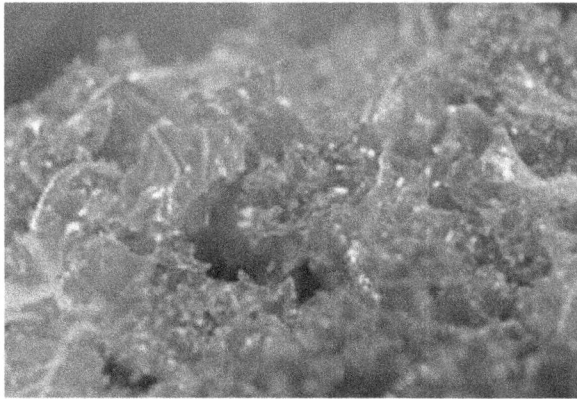

SWEET POTATO FRIES

- 3 medium sweet potatoes
- 1 tsp. fresh rosemary, chopped
- 1 tbsp. olive oil

- 1/4 tsp. olive oil

Instructions:

1. Preheat oven to 180 degrees.
2. Scrub potatoes and cut length ways into desired chip thickness.
3. In a bowl combine olive oil, sea salt, and rosemary.
4. Place chips on a tray lined with baking paper and coat with the olive oil mixture.
5. Place in oven and cook for around 30 – 35 minutes, turning once in cooking time.

Once cooked remove and sprinkle with sea salt. Nice served with a fresh tomato salsa sauce.

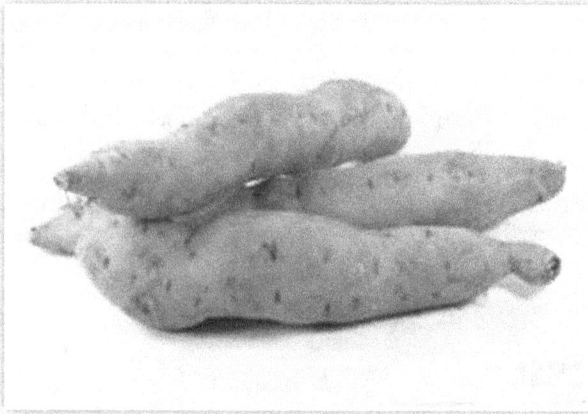

Desserts

BANANA CAKES

- 3 large or 4 medium overripe bananas
- 3 eggs
- 3 tbsp extra virgin coconut oil
- 1 tbsp honey
- 1 tsp vanilla
- 1/3 cup coconut flour
- 1/3 cup arrowroot powder

Instructions

Blend together and bake at 190 for 35 - 40min.

CHIA SEED PUDDING

- Pour bowl of coconut cream. Add 1 tsp. chia seeds. Place in refrigerator. Chill for an hour, and then serve.

JAM

- Soak any dried fruit in water for a minimum of 30 minutes. Using a blender, blitz on high for a few minutes until it thickens, then store in a glass jar with a tight lid.

JAM PIE

- Puree dates and almonds to use as a base. Press into pan. Combine jam with gelatin. Pour filling into base and freeze for 30 minutes.

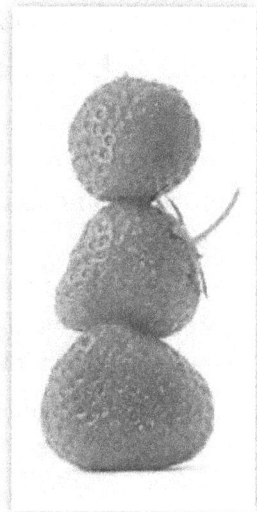

LEMON BLISS BALLS

- Dates, pureed
- Puffed quinoa
- Coconut flakes
- ¼ cup melted cacao butter
- Whole lemon

Mix. Form into ball and roll in shredded coconut.

CHOCOLATE PROTEIN BALLS

- 1 cup nuts and seeds of choice
- 4 fresh dates
- 2 tbl raw organic honey
- 1 tbl Protein Powder
- Shredded coconut or grated dark chocolate

Instructions:

1. Combine in food processor and roll into balls.
2. Roll into shredded coconut or grated dark chocolate to coat.
3. Store in the fridge in an airtight container.

RAW FOODS CHOCOLATE MOUSSE

- Avocados are good for a simple chocolate mousse. Simply blend avocado, cacao, and honey. Chill.

GLUTEN FREE COCONUT RAISIN COOKIES

- 1/4 cup grapeseed oil
- 1/4 cup agave nectar
- 1 tsp vanilla extract
- 1 1/4 cups blanched almond flour
- 1/4 teaspoon celtic sea salt
- 1/4 teaspoon baking soda
- 1/2 cup walnuts, toasted and chopped
- 1/2 cup coconut, shredded
- 1/4 cup raisins

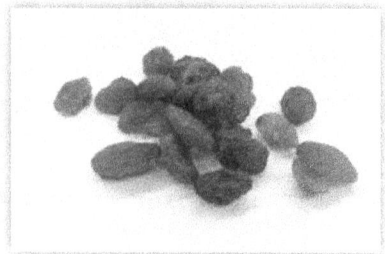

Instructions:

1. In a large bowl, combine oil, agave and vanilla.

2. In a medium bowl, combine almond flour salt, baking soda, walnuts, coconut and raisins.

3. Stir dry ingredients into wet, mixing thoroughly.

4. Form dough into 1 inch balls and flatten onto a parchment lined baking sheet.

5. Bake at 350° for 8-10 minutes, until golden brown around the edges.

6. Cool and serve.

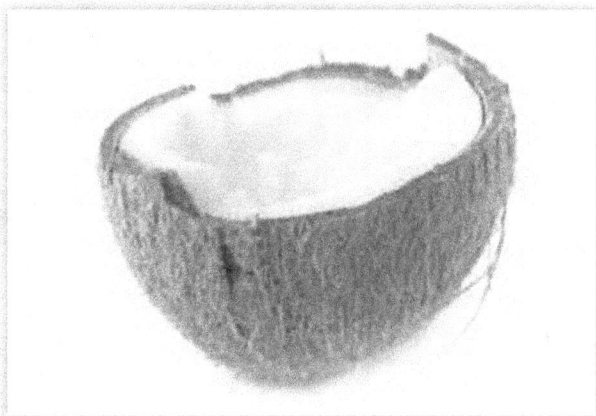

APPENDIX C

AMINO ACID—ANY ONE OF many acids that occur naturally in living things and that include some which form proteins.

Carbohydrate—any one of various substances found in certain foods (such as bread, rice, and potatoes) that provide your body with heat and energy and are made of carbon, hydrogen, and oxygen.

Coeliac disease—a chronic hereditary intestinal disorder in which an inability to absorb the gliadin portion of gluten results in the gliadin triggering an immune response that damages the intestinal mucosa; also celiac sprue.

Composting—a mixture that consists largely of decayed organic matter and is used for fertilizing and conditioning land.

Ferment/Fermented—a living organism (as a yeast) that causes fermentation by virtue of its enzymes. Added: The bacteria produced by fermentation aids in digestion.

Hormones—a product of living cells that circulates in body fluids (as blood) or sap and produces a specific often stimulatory effect on the activity of cells usually remote from its point of origin.

Legume—the fruit or seed of plants of the legume family (as peas or beans) used for food.

pH—a measure of acidity and alkalinity of a solution that is a number on a scale on which a value of 7 represents neutrality and lower numbers indicate increasing acidity and higher numbers increasing alkalinity and on which each unit of change represents a tenfold change in acidity or alkalinity and that is the negative logarithm of the effective hydrogen-ion concentration or hydrogen-ion activity in gram equivalents per liter of the solution; also : the condition represented by a pH number

Protein—any of various naturally occurring extremely complex substances that consist of amino-acid residues joined by peptide bonds, contain the elements carbon, hydrogen, nitrogen, oxygen, usually sulfur, and occasionally other elements (as phosphorus or iron), and include many essential biological compounds (as enzymes, hormones, or antibodies) .

SCOBY—Acronym for 'symbiotic colony of bacteria and yeast' which is a culture used to create kombucha.

Sprouts—edible sprouts especially from recently germinated seeds (as of alfalfa or mung beans).

All definitions provided courtesy of Merriam Webster at *http://www. merriam-webster.com/dictionary/* .

CITATIONS

[1] Pappas, Stephanie. "Optimism Boosts Immune System.".com. TechMedia Network, 25 Mar. 2010. Web. 01 Sept. 2013. <http://www.livescience.com/8158-optimism-boosts-immune-system.html>.

[2] Beling, Stephanie. (1997). Power Foods: Good Food, Good Health with Phytochemicals, Nature's Own Energy boosters. The role of positive affect. Psychological Science, 21(3), 448-55.

[3] Mercola, Dr. Joseph. "The Toxic Import from China Hidden in This Everyday Beverage..." Mercola.com. Dr. Mercola, n.d. Web. <http://articles.mercola.com/sites/articles/archive/2011/10/11/dr-bill-osmunson-on-fluoride.aspx>.

[4] Berry, Sarah. "'I Can Take Any Diet and Tear It Apart'" The Sydney Morning Herald. Sydney Morning Herald, 15 May 2013. Web. 29 Aug. 2013.

[5] Cann, Kevin. "Nutrition and Depression." The Paleo Diet Robb Wolf on Paleolithic Nutrition Intermittent Fasting and Fitness RSS. Robb Wolf, 23 Mar. 2012. Web. 29 Aug. 2013.

[6] Dinan, Timothy G. "Cytokines and Their Effect on Serotonin." Current Opinion in Psychiatry 22 (2009): 32-36. Medscape. Medscape, 2009. Web. 29 Aug. 2013. <http://www.medscape.com/viewarticle/584794_7>.

[7] Visser, J., Rozing, J., Sapone, A., Lammers, K. and Fasano, A. (2009), Tight Junctions, Intestinal Permeability, and Autoimmunity. Annals of the New York Academy of Sciences, 1165:–205. doi:.1111/j.1749-6632.2009.04037.x

[8] Jenny. "Against the Grain. 10 Reasons to Give Up Grains." Nourished Kitchen. Nourished Kitchen, 1 May 2009. Web. 29 Aug. 2013. <http://nourishedkitchen.com/against-the-grain-10-reasons-to-give-up-grains/>.

[9] Consalvo, Dana. "Serotonin: The Feel Good Hormone - The Toonari Post - News, Powered by the People!" The Toonari Post News Powered by the People Serotonin The Feel Good Hormone Comments. Toonari Post, 12 Apr. 2011. Web. 29 Aug. 2013. <http://www.toonaripost.com/2011/04/us-news/serotonin-the-feel-good-hormone/>.

[10] Hadhazy, Adam. "Think Twice: How the Gut's "Second Brain" Influences Mood and Well-Being: Scientific American." Scientific American. Georg Von Holtzbrinck Publishing Group, 12 Feb. 2010. Web. 29 Aug. 2013. <http://www.scientificamerican.com/article.cfm?id=gut-second-brain>.

[11] Huebner, FR, KW Lieberman, RP Rubino, and JS Wall. "Demonstration of High Opioid-like Activity in Isolated Peptides from Wheat Gluten Hydrolysates." US National Library of Medicine National Institute of Health (1984): 1139-147. National Center for Biotechnology Information. U.S. National Library of Medicine, Nov.-Dec. 1984. Web. 29 Aug. 2013. <*http:// www.ncbi.nlm.nih.gov/pubmed/6099562*>.

[12] Rodriguez, R.H.N., Vanessa. "5 Liver Health Tips for Weight Loss." *Active.com*. The Active Network, Inc., n.d. Web. 30 Aug. 2013.

[13] "Protein."NHMRC Nutrient Reference Values. Australian Government: National Health and Medical Research Council, n.d. Web. 06 Oct. 2013.

[14] Magee, MPH, RDWeb, Elaine. "Good Carbs, Bad Carbs: Understanding Natural and Refined Carbohydrates." WebMD. WebMD, n.d. Web. 30 Aug. 2013.

[15] "Obesity in Australia | MODI."in Australia | MODI. Monash Obesity and Diabetes Institute, 6 Aug. 2013. Web. 19 Oct. 2013.

[16] Snyder, Kimberly. "The Difference in How Fructose and Glucose Affect Your Body."*Kimberly Snyder The Difference in How Fructose and Glucose Affect Your Body.* Kimberly Snyder's Health & Beauty Detox, n.d. Web. 20 Oct. 2013.

[17] "Health Benefits of Coconut Oil."Facts. Organic Information Services Pvt Ltd., n.d. Web. 31 Aug. 2013. <*http://www.organicfacts.net/organic-oils/organic-coconut-oil/health-benefits-of-coconut-oil.html*>.

[18] "Vitamins and Minerals."Choices. *Gov.UK*, 26 Nov. 2012. Web. 31 Aug. 2013. <*http://www.nhs.uk/Conditions/vitamins-minerals/Pages/vitamins-minerals.aspx*>.

[19] "Minerals: MedlinePlus."S National Library of Medicine. U.S. National Library of Medicine, 17 June 2013. Web. 31 Aug. 2013. <*http://www.nlm.nih.gov/medlineplus/minerals.html*>.

[20] Warburg, Otto H. "The Prime Cause and Prevention of Cancer, by Dr. Otto Warburg."LIBRARY -. AlkalizeForHealth, n.d. Web. 31 Aug. 2013.

[21] Bridgeford, Ross. "What Is Acidosis – The Problem of an Acidic Lifestyle."Alkaline Diet Blog RSS. N.p., n.d. Web. 01 Sept. 2013. <*http://www.energiseforlife.com/wordpress/2006/08/08/what-is-acidosis-the-problem-of-an-acidic-lifestyle/*>.

[22] "Chemicals in Meat Cooked at High Temperatures and Cancer Risk."*National Cancer Institute at the National Institutes of Health*. National Cancer Institute, 15 Oct. 2010. Web. 12 Oct. 2013.

[23] Torres, Marco. "Student's Experiment Shows How Microwaved Water Kills Plants After Just Days." Student's Experiment Shows How Microwaved Water Kills Plants After Just Days. *PreventDisease.com*, 17 Apr. 2012. Web. 29 Aug. 2013.

[24] Mercola, Joseph. "Why Did the Russians Ban an Appliance Found in 90% of American Homes?" *Mercola.com*-Take Control of Your Health. N.p., 18 May 2010. Web.<*http://articles.mercola. com/sites/articles/archive/2010/05/18/microwave-hazards.aspx*>

[25] Baby Center Medical Advisory Board. "How Breastfeeding Benefits You and Your Baby." BabyCenter. Baby Center LLC, n.d. Web. 30 Aug. 2013.

[26] "Benefits of Breastfeeding for Mom." *HealthyChildren.org*. American Academy of Pediatrics, 11 May 2013. Web. 30 Aug. 2013.

[27] Becker, Eve. "Soy Controversy." Living Without. Living Without, Inc., Oct.-Nov. 2010. Web. 30 Aug. 2013. <*http://www.livingwithout.com/issues/4_10/soy_controversy-2180-1.html*>.

[28] Mercola, Dr. Joseph. "ALERT: Food Toxins Found in Baby Formula." *Mercola.com* -Take Control of Your Health. N.p., 25 Oct. 2011. Web. 30 Aug. 2013. *<http://articles.mercola.com/sites/articles/archive/2011/10/25/toxins-in-baby-formula-milk.aspx>.*

[29] Wolf, Nicki. "The Advantages of Using Organic Baby Formula." SFGate: Home Guides. Demand Media, n.d. Web. 30 Aug. 2013.

[30] "What Is Organic Gardening? What Does It Mean to Be an Organic Gardener?" *What Is Organic Gardening and Why Should I Care?: Organic Gardening.* Rodale Inc., n.d. Web. 03 Sept. 2013. *<http://www.organicgardening.com/learn-and-grow/what-*is-organic-gardening>.

[31] "Natural Fermentation: Salt vs. Whey vs. Starter Cultures." Cultures for Health. N.p., *n.d.* Web. 05 Sept. 2013.

[32] "Sprouts Have The Highest Concentration Of Nutrition Per Calorie Of Any Food." *Healthy Eating Advisor.* The Healthy Eating Advisor, n.d. Web. 05 Sept. 2013.

[33] "The Basics of Composting." *The Garden Of Oz.* N.p., n.d. Web. 06 Sept. 2013.

AUTHOR BIO:
Samantha Baird

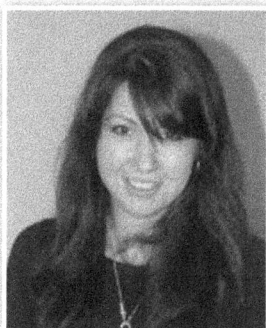

AUTHOR, SAMANTHA BAIRD, IS a certified Food Coach. She completed her Cert IV training at the Food Coach Institute and is currently pursuing a raw food certification at The Health Arts college, as well as studying raw food certification with David Wolfe at Body Mind Institute.

Samantha—known as Sam by her clients—also completed an online certification of natural health with Natural Choices, and has enrolled to complete her advanced diploma in nutritional medicine in 2014.

Sam originally started her career as a hairdresser. She struggled with health issues and suffered through two miscarriages. She first became interested in nutrition and healthy living when her youngest daughter, as a newborn, began struggling with major health problems due to great difficulty in digesting her food. Realizing something was very wrong, Sam's desire to help her daughter inspired her to dig into holistic nutrition. Her studies helped her to see and understand the drastic health impacts she had already experienced herself due to her job, as she was required to handle toxic materials.

Her knowledge took her on a new course, and she became a qualified Food Coach. After implementing critical dietary changes for her and her family, her little girl is now happy, healthy, and a sound sleeper—and Sam is 19kg lighter!

Sam is living out her new passion as a Food Coach by utilizing her newfound mission and goals:

- Her mission is to help educate others on how to sustain a primal lifestyle
- Her goal is to give you personalized service by discovering your health needs, guiding you through the learning curve, and helping you build positive health habits for the future

Join her at *http://www.food4health.com.au* and start your health journey together!